HEAL NOW

OTHER BOOKS BY ROBIN H. MILLER, MD

Invisible or Invincible: Your Choice
by Robin H. Miller, MD
Triune Integrative Medicine, 2022

Healed! Health & Wellness for the 21st Century:
Wisdom, Secrets, and Fun Straight From the Leading Edge
by Robin H. Miller, MD and David Es. Kahn, MS CPT
Triune Integrative Medicine, 2017

Kids Ask The Doctor
by Robin H. Miller, MD
Triune Integrative Medicine, 2016

The Smart Woman's Guide to Midlife and Beyond:
A No Nonsense Approach to Staying Healthy After 50
By Robin Miller, MD and Janet Horn, MD
New Harbinger Publications, 2008

HEAL NOW

*Time to Un-sick Yourself
with the
21st Century Guide to Wellness*

ROBIN H. MILLER, MD, MHS

TRIUNE INTEGRATIVE MEDICINE
2023

Published by Triune Integrative Medicine
Medford, Oregon

https://www.triunemed.com

Print ISBN: 979-8-218-21846-1
Ebook ISBN: 979-8-218-21936-9

Book design by
Lucky Valley Press
www.luckyvalleypress.com

Printed in the USA on acid-free paper

DEDICATION

I dedicate this book to my patients, who have been my greatest teachers, and to my mother, who has inspired me to be as healthy as I can be!

CONTENTS

The Issues • Navigating the System • Good Service Accessibility •
Quality of Care • Expense • Relying On a Broken System • Integrative
Medicine • Be Organized/Be Open/Be Honest/Be Ready to Change

Part One
Smarts, Hearts & Farts,
The Integration of the Brain, Heart, and Gut
The Brain and the Heart • The Gut and the Heart
The Heart and the Brain

The Brain 101 • The Brain Gut Connection • Alzheimer's Disease
• Parkinson's Disease • TBI Traumatic Brain Injury • The Wrap Up

Heart 101 • The Heart Gut Connection • The Vagus Nerve as the
Wanderer • How to Save a Life (Your Own) • Evaluate Your Risk •
Risk Factors You Can Change • What About Stroke? • The Wrap Up

Gut 101 • IBS Irritable Bowel Syndrome • Allergies/Lactose Intolerance
• Fructose Intolerance • Gluten Intolerance • Celiac Disease • True
Food Allergies • Cranky Bowels • MTHFR Mutations • IBD/Colon
Cancer • Bacterial Overgrowth • When All Your Tests Are Negative •
Trust Your Gut • Prebiotics, Probiotics, and the Microbiome • Exercise
• Inflammation and the Gut • The Wrap Up

Part Two
Stay Alive and Thrive
To My Younger Self
Back to Reality

Part Three
Make It a Practice
No Excuses: Make *You* a Daily Priority

"They who have health have hope;
and they who have hope, have everything."
– Maya Angelou

PROLOGUE

In February 2017, *Healed: Health and Wellness for the 21st Century* was published, with the subtitle: *Wisdom, Secrets, and Fun Straight from the Leading Edge.* At that time, my coauthor Dave Kahn (a teacher and certified personal trainer) and I wanted to make readers aware of the fun, secrets, and major benefits of ballroom dancing. We had been inspired by an article published in the New England Journal of Medicine in 2003 entitled, "Leisure activities and the risk of dementia in the elderly."

The study noted that the risk of dementia was decreased by 76% in those who did ballroom dance twice weekly[1]. Dave and I are avid dancers and wanted to open our readers' eyes (and minds) to the exciting possibilities. The book's focus was on utilizing dance for the healing and prevention of diseases ranging from high blood pressure to Alzheimer's disease. And dance does have that power.

Since the book was published five years ago, much has changed. We have experienced a major pandemic and witnessed the collapse of our medical healthcare system. And while ballroom dance is a powerful aid to health and healing, there is so much more to share—things we didn't know five years ago. In this book, the advice and information have been expanded to include more opportunities for you to *become* and *stay* healthy.

The research and information in the chapters to come will give you a roadmap to health and healing. I am proud and excited to introduce you to *Heal Now – Time to Un-sick Yourself with the 21st Century Guide to Wellness.* You can read the book straight through or pick and choose the chapters that interest you. Whichever method you choose, I hope you will be inspired, find tremendous benefit, *and* become the healthiest version of YOU.

— *Robin H. Miller, MD*

• • •

The one and only person
who is going to keep you healthy
is YOU.

• • •

PARTNERS IN WELLNESS

The one and only person who is going to keep you healthy is YOU. Your doctor won't. The healthcare system won't. Big Pharma *definitely* won't. While medical science has advanced by leaps and bounds just in my lifetime, the expected payoff for patients is not there.

In fact, a child born in the US is 76% more likely to die before their first birthday than babies born in other wealthy countries. (Don't even get me started on the maternal mortality rate.) If the baby survives infancy, they have a 57% greater likelihood of dying before they reach adulthood when compared to babies of other wealthy countries. This is due to poverty rates, lack of education, a weak social safety net, and lack of prenatal care. When mothers do not receive prenatal care, they are three times more likely to have a low-birthweight baby, and the infant mortality rate increases five times for these babies.[1]

For adults, the average life expectancy in the US dropped in 2020 and declined further in 2022 due to the ongoing drug epidemic, poverty, and the COVID-19 pandemic. Overall, it has gone from 77 years in 2020 to 76.4 years in 2021. For women, the average life expectancy went from 79.9 years in 2020 to 79.1 in 2021, and for men from 74.2 years in 2020 to 73.2 years in 2021.[2] Granted, many factors are at play. A medical system overwhelmed by acutely ill patients discouraging those in need of preventive or follow-up care, poor access, and the potential for insanely high medical bills all contribute to the problem.

I have seen those needing relatively urgent cardiac procedures put on waiting lists hundreds of patients long. Some needed cancer evaluations and were still delayed by weeks or months, and others simply were told they could not be evaluated due to a lack of providers. Those who go to the emergency room wait for hours, sometimes days. If they need to be admitted, there are often no beds. Patients are placed in hallways with lines between stretchers. It's reminiscent of third-world medicine, and we Americans live in one of the wealthiest countries in the world.

Advancements and capabilities are improving, but outcomes aren't improving at the same rate. Doctors are great at saving a life (most of the time) but not at keeping you out of the hospital. Harold Thimbleby, a professor at Swansea University, says it best in "Technology and the Future of Healthcare:"

> *Pluck a nurse and surgeon out of the nineteenth century and transport them into a modern 21st-century hospital and it would be a thoroughly recognizable place, with the same hierarchies and strict cultures. Patients are treated as helpless, stripped of their clothes and possessions, lying in beds, and almost completely ignorant of their illnesses. They might be disappointed in our treatment, particularly of old people, but I don't think it would surprise them.*[3]

There have been remarkable changes to medicine and its practice in the last fifty years. Technologically, we have advanced by leaps and bounds. But, as far as the practice of medicine goes, I agree with Harold Thimbleby. It feels as if we have gone back into the dark ages. Medical professionals' reliance on technology is so great that for most the art of medicine has been lost. Computed tomography (CT) scans have replaced neurologic exams. Blood tests have replaced patient histories and observations. Supplements have replaced healthy diets. Technology is great but loses its power when the patient is left out of the equation.

The Only Person Who Can Keep You Healthy

We all need doctors when something acute is going on or we need preventive strategies, but the one and only person who is going to keep you healthy is YOU. You *must* become your best partner in wellness.

We can no longer depend on the medical system to be invested in our health. The reasons for this are varied and have been increasing and accelerating for years. We have a system that for years has fostered dependence on "the doctor" to evaluate and treat us. Slowly, almost imperceptibly, patient responsibility has gone by the wayside. And of course, it has! We feel we need that MRI to make our backs feel better. It is a test, not a treatment. We want that fancy stress test to make our hearts feel better. (Again, it is a test, not a treatment.) Those who are overweight or obese may desire a knee replacement to make their pain better when, for many, just losing five pounds will take the pressure off and reduce their pain, and there is no longer a need for the invasive procedure. Diabetics crave that fancy blood sugar monitor to improve their diabetes. (The monitor isn't going to do that, YOU are.) Tempting as it is to punt responsibility to our providers and all their cool tech, each of us is solely responsible for our health.

Maybe the best way to see why it is *so* important for all of us to understand the issues is to share my observations and experiences throughout my career. I have seen amazing (and sometimes horrifying) changes that have altered my perspective, surprising even me.

The Evolution

I went to medical school in the late 70s. When I started my internship in internal medicine, there were no CT scans or advanced imaging; instead, we had to use the power of observation and physical diagnosis. The lifesaving procedures we rely on today were not available back then. People with heart disease died without the benefit of stents, bypass surgery, and angiograms. Throughout my training, I developed an interest in preventive cardiology and studied families at high risk for heart disease. At the time, it was a foregone conclusion that you would die young if you had a strong family history and risk factors such as abnormally high cholesterol.

I spent three years at Johns Hopkins Hospital researching diet and exercise and the effect of risk factor modification on heart disease. We helped patients and their families eat healthier and exercise regularly to decrease their chances of dying of heart disease. I continued research and teaching at SUNY Stony Brook in New York. Around that time, the obesity epidemic had not hit yet, and I felt like we were making headway with the people we treated. What I found, however, was that the more I became involved in research, the more I missed patient care. It is funny how when one gets deep into research, the individual patients seem to be less important than the overall concept of helping population groups. Sadly, it took away my focus on direct patient care, and that didn't sit well with me.

Patient care, it turns out, was my real passion. When I moved away from research and moved across the country to Oregon with my family in 1991, I was again seeing people and enjoying taking care of them. That was the time when things shifted in medicine. The obesity epidemic took off. Obesity increased from 12% in 1991 to 17.9% in 1998.[4] Unfortunately, the epidemic has kept on growing…and so have the waistbands of the US population.

I joined a group practice in Medford, Oregon. The environment was great to work in at the time. But again, the winds were shifting, and the attitudes of physicians and patients were changing. I distinctly remember meeting with my colleagues and discussing how important it was for patients to exercise and be on a heart-healthy diet. At the end of my talk, one of the distinguished cardiologists got up and commented that we no longer had to worry about that. Statin drugs had just come out and were being prescribed regularly to lower cholesterol. He said patients could eat their Twinkies and take a statin without an issue. Problem solved—NOT.

To say I was appalled would be an understatement. It was a foreshadowing of what nightmares were to come. People seemed to no longer care about what they ate, relying on a statin to manage cholesterol for them; diabetic patients checked out of their diet treatment and blood sugar monitoring, assuming metformin would keep everything under control. Physicians were no longer taking the time to talk to their patients, opting instead to write out a few scripts. "Do you have a problem? There's a pill for that!" became a pervasive mindset among doctors and patients alike. It's how we have ended up in such a "sick" state.

When the time was ripe for improving people's lives with the incredible development of technology, such as coronary artery bypass and imaging techniques using Magnetic Resonance Imaging (MRI) and CT scans, our ability to help patients with essentials such as healthy lifestyle choices were being hampered. The practice I had been enjoying became a mill. I was expected to see patients every ten minutes and do physicals and intakes in twenty minutes. There was NO time to talk. Insurance companies were driving us to be more efficient, and management demanded we be more productive to bring in more money. Patients were falling through the cracks in a bureaucracy that has only become more out of control with time.

Medication after medication was developed to treat everything from depression to erectile dysfunction. Little by little, with the help of Big Pharma and physicians being pushed to the max, patient responsibility went out the window. I was beside myself. I went into medicine to help people, to listen and assess, and then come up with a plan. That is not what happened. *So, I quit.*

I had reached my limit. I went to the head of the clinic, said, "I quit," and walked out. I enrolled in an integrative medicine fellowship with Dr. Andrew Weil in Arizona and went back to the basics. I was able to hone my listening skills and found the compassion and empathy that had been buried by my inability to act on them in ten-minute visits.

If this is how it felt from a physician's perspective, imagine how a patient feels! The system is so much worse for patients than it is for doctors. After multiple short non-productive visits, it would be easy for patients to feel helpless and see the medical system as adversarial. It is all too easy for patients to "check out" when it comes to being responsible for their health and feel hopeless and victimized. I wanted to offer a different, healthier and more productive opportunity for health and wellness, and that meant making my patients my number one priority.

Medicine Practiced in a New Way

I started my own clinic that did not rely on insurance, which gave me more freedom to practice medicine the way I'd always imagined it to be. I could spend ninety minutes with new patients and sixty minutes with those having a yearly physical. We had plenty of time to tackle multiple issues, answer questions, and have deeper discussions about their health. I was happier, and my patients were delighted. Yes, it cost more than a copay, but when people considered their health's importance, the money out of pocket was worth it. In addition, if you are paying out of your own funds, you are far more likely to work with someone to improve your health!

I practice integrative medicine. *What is that?* you ask. It is a patient-focused approach where the doctor and patient are a team. Before, I chased diseases for people and got nowhere. With integrative medicine, I could get to the bottom of what was happening with them. More than that, I got to know my patients as the people they are. My questions were unlike any you're used to hearing from your primary care physician: *How did you grow up? What formed your health habits? What traumas may have contributed?* I made it a point to get to the heart of my patients' stories. These things are as integral to their health and well-being as labs and vital signs.

Through this approach, I have seen profound changes in overweight patients. After countless diets, they never seem to lose and often gain even more weight. I realized that when we talked about their past, the reasons why they were overeating became apparent. Many were molested or raped. Unconsciously, the extra weight was a protective shield. Therapy with a psychologist often worked wonders, and those patients have maintained a healthy weight.

Many with recurrent gut issues that cause severe distress have underlying emotional experiences causing the problems. Past traumas ranging from physical attacks to fires causing loss of their homes and the death of a loved one can all contribute. Again, psychological evaluation and treatment and someone who has partnered with them to truly understand and listen to them has made all the difference and allowed them to heal.

By listening and digging deep, I have found medical problems I have only read about. Periodic paralysis, where patients literally wilt due to potassium level imbalances; a weird benign tumor of the chest called a teratoma, a tumor containing hair, muscle and often bone; hidden adrenal tumors (pheochromocytoma) giving off hormone surges creating a physiological response that appears like panic attacks. Most of these patients were written off as crazy by doctors without the time and interest to get to the root of the patient's problems.

For me, the relationships I create with patients are vital. Intellectually, I enjoy the challenge of resolving what is going on. Emotionally, it is gratifying to truly help people and connect. That said, I have had to learn how to temper that enthusiasm and not get carried away.

At first, I tried to participate in my patients' healing too much! I was enabling them. I remember calling patients to remind them to take a walk. I even found these talking cards where you can record your voice, and it speaks when the card is opened. I would record myself saying "Step away from the refrigerator NOW!" or "Turn around, put your walking shoes on, and get out the door!" and have them put it on their refrigerator to remind them to keep away until mealtime! The cards were fun, though they weren't all that effective. But then, I had an eye-opening experience that helped me shift gears. Bear with me and indulge me while I digress. You will see where I am going with this.

In addition to being a practicing physician, I am a medical reporter. I was fortunate to be able to do a story on horse therapy in 2004. A wonderful psychologist named June Gunter Ed.D. had several specially trained horses that were used for psychotherapy. For the news story, I followed the program just as her clients would. First, she had me brush the horse named Rocky. I was going as fast as possible, and she suggested I slow down and do it mindfully. Then, she had me get in the ring with him. It was just Rocky and me.

• • •

"How am I gonna do that?"

• • •

"Okay, now I want you to get Rocky to move around the ring. A full circle."

I looked up at this giant horse, looked back at June, and said, "How am I gonna do that?"

June simply smiled at me and said, "With your intention. That's how."

So, armed with my intentions, I started jumping up and down and running around, doing anything I could think of to get Rocky to take a step. All I did was wear myself out. I was so tired that I had no choice but to slow down and connect energetically with the horse. Then lo and behold, he ran around the ring.

June pointed out that I needed to be more mindful and reminded me that while I could get the horse to move, I was doing all the work. She wondered how this translated to my family and my practice. That was a tremendous insight because I am a *doer* and always have been. I was trying so hard and doing everything for everyone, and it was helping no one.

HEAL NOW

When I was doing the work for my patients, I was enabling them and unconsciously telling them they couldn't do it on their own. Treating people as if they are weak doesn't help and can hinder them. They can make the changes, but they need to trust themselves to be responsible for their choices and health. And I needed to have faith in them.

Since then, I have met most people halfway. I no longer call my patients to remind them to get out and exercise. However, I will refer them to inexpensive trainers I know will help. I won't give them talking cards, but I will suggest they check out local groups to help them with their menu planning and cooking. For emotional support, I have found people in our area with affordable innovative programs for help and support. I now realize my job is not to be an enabler; I need to be a partner.

• • •

80% of chronic disease is due to lifestyle choices.

• • •

What I am driving at is that there is only one person who can heal you, and that is you. The opposite is also true: no one can do a better job of killing you slowly than YOU. We all need to be aware that 80% of chronic disease is due to lifestyle choices.[5] Let me say this again... *Eighty percent of chronic disease is due to unhealthy lifestyle choices.* You have a choice.

This concept has fueled my search to step out of the medical practice box (and sometimes get rid of it altogether) and find new, innovative ways to help people heal themselves and be well. Sometimes it requires going back to basics, and other times I have ventured into the wild world of new science, such as the exploding field of genetics and microbiology. Over the years, I have learned so much and found simple but impactful ways to help patients. Now it's time to share these ideas.

The truth is, you have tremendous power in the trajectory of your health and the quality of your life. You have more agency than you might think, more than you may have been made to feel by the medical establishment. There is no need to feel like a victim when you can be a partner instead. You may need to grow a pair and be forceful (nicely, of course!), but you are your best advocate. You know yourself better than anyone else. You know what will work for you. The key is to find someone who can help you. An integrative medicine provider is such a person. (More on that in a moment.)

• • •

Nothing tastes better than being alive!

• • •

Revamping your health is simple, but it isn't easy. Change is hard, but it can be done. Often it means stepping outside of your comfort zone. And that's where the resistance—and the excuses—come in. And believe me, I've heard them all! I remember a patient with type 2 diabetes who ate double chocolate glazed donuts regularly. I told her she needed to cut out the donuts, and the notion of that was unfathomable to her. She just couldn't do it. How sad. Nothing tastes better than being alive!

Another patient had retinal bleeding in the back of his eye. He is diabetic, and this bleeding is not unusual for those with diabetes as the disease progresses. Still, he refused to check his daily blood sugars, claiming he was way too busy. Doing what, I am not sure, given that he is retired. I asked him how he felt about going blind if his diabetes was left unchecked, but he was in total denial. You are not too busy to prevent blindness!

I had a female patient with gallbladder disease. I suggested that if she avoided fat in her diet, she could avoid surgery for her gallbladder problem. She couldn't give up her daily French fries and ended up in surgery eventually. Are French fries worth it?

I have another patient with something called Barrett's esophagus. This is a precancerous condition of the esophagus that causes painful ulcerations. The treatment is an acid blocker that can help prevent it from becoming cancerous. This patient refused to take the medication because she feared the potential side effects due to poor absorption of certain minerals such as calcium and magnesium. These side effects could be overcome by switching to calcium citrate, which is absorbed in the absence of stomach acid, and adding magnesium. But she didn't do it. Unfortunately, her esophageal condition did not improve, and she needed an invasive procedure to treat it.

• • •

Minor side effects do not trump cancer!

• • •

The best excuse utilizes what I call the Scarlett O'Hara approach to health. For those of you too young to have seen the movie, *Gone with the Wind*, the main character Scarlett O'Hara, puts off thinking about difficult things. She always says, "I'll think about that tomorrow." That is precisely what many of us do. We will think about changing our eating and health habits or exercise habits... tomorrow.

My father-in-law, Jerry, gave some of the best advice about life, health, and business. He said there are three essential things:

Be on time. Write it down. Do it now.

DO IT NOW is something I think about often. For your health, it is essential. Because if nothing changes, nothing changes. And that's why I wrote *Heal Now.* Being accountable and responsible for your health will save your life. It will improve and prolong the quality and duration of your life. As a doctor, I am so frustrated by what I see because I care about what happens to all of us, doctors *and* patients.

The Issues

I am the last person I expected to write a book like this. But as a doctor, I am so disappointed in our medical establishment. There are a multitude of things that have gone wonky.

You can't navigate the system. So much healthcare management is done on the computer, from appointments to follow-ups. And while this can be expeditious, it can also be exclusionary to those unfamiliar with using such software. During the pandemic, many seniors were left out in the cold when COVID-19 vaccine appointments had to be made online and they could not navigate the system. Even now, getting results utilizing the various "My Charts" is confusing and alienating.

You can't find good service. Where does it state that the doctor's time is more important than a patient's time? And yet, it is not unusual to wait an hour in the waiting room for an appointment. How hard would it be to call someone and say the doctor is running late? One office in our area cancels your appointment if you arrive ten minutes late, but they give you nothing if the doctor makes you wait fifty to sixty minutes to be seen. Personally, I think it should be "no charge" for the visit!

Accessibility is difficult. Even when something is semi-emergent, getting in to see someone can be impossible. Primary care doctors are retiring in droves. Just when you find a new doctor, they are gone, and the clinics do not offer an alternative. This has been particularly challenging for seniors on Medicare, and it can be downright deadly for those on chronic pain management because they need someone to refill their prescriptions. They can get very ill or die if they go into acute withdrawal due to no medications.

Quality of care is often poor. As we discussed earlier, doctors are often rushed and stressed. They don't have the time to explain things well, and miscommunications often result in errors or patients not getting the medications they need. Poor communication can also lead to worse care down the line, as patients may not understand the next steps or arrange proper follow-ups and referrals.

Medical care (good or bad) is insanely expensive. Doctor visits are costly, and the medications are even more expensive. I have seen too many patients have essential treatments prescribed and then be unable to buy them due to costs. They don't want to bother their doctors, so they simply don't take them. There are usually cheaper alternatives or ways around the expense with special compassionate funds. Still, you have to know they exist to get them—and when communication breaks down between a doctor and patient, these resources go unmentioned.

These issues are only going to get worse. Doctors are so burned out post-COVID, and patients are seeing more physician assistants and nurse practitioners. There may be advantages to this since they tend to be more thorough. However, the depth of knowledge is not there, and doctors offer a more comprehensive look and evaluation for patients with complicated histories.

You don't want to have to rely on this system, and you want to avoid needing it if possible. Fortunately, there is a lot you can do. And that's what this book is about. By being a good partner in wellness, you can revamp your health and have a completely new understanding of what you can do to improve your health outcomes. This isn't just about keeping you out of the hospital. You can sharpen your mind, fire up your sex life, and feel better than ever, regardless of how old you are and where your baseline health is right now. It is never too late.

• • •

As my father-in-law would say, "DO IT NOW!"

• • •

In days of yore, the classic family doctors (like Marcus Welby, MD, I know he is a fantasy doctor, but still…) might have taken care of all your health needs for you; but I have news for you, that isn't going to happen today. Our medical system is broken, and the COVID-19 pandemic has shown us just how badly.

Doctors, if you can see them, are overworked and burned out. Telemedicine is available but is not a good substitute for in-person visits. Emergency rooms are overwhelmed in our state by drug overdoses and homeless people. There is a delay in caring for diseases that can be prevented or treated early. Many feel hopeless, but that does not have to be the case.

There are times when you need a doctor. There are instances when things go awry. I get that. However, when eighty percent of disease is due to lifestyle choices, there is so much that we, as individuals, can do. This book will help you feel empowered and motivated to improve your health and make the changes you need to reach your maximum health potential. It is not meant to replace your doctor, but it may keep you from needing one! See yourself as your primary partner in health. When you do need a doctor, I suggest you choose an integrative medicine physician or at least someone who listens.

• • •

Integrative medicine practitioners find ways
to help patients heal on their own.

• • •

What Do I Mean by Integrative Medicine?

When I speak to groups of people about this, many will invariably come up to me afterward and say what I am suggesting is impossible. However, a growing field of medicine is spreading throughout the country: integrative medicine.

Integrative medicine is focused on the *patient*. (What a concept!) The provider partners with the patient to promote wellness in the mind, body, and spirit. In doing so, the patient will become healthy and stay well, and disease will be prevented. Conversely, most medicine these days is disease oriented. A patient presents with a problem, and that problem gets treated. Little time is spent looking at the whole picture and getting to the root of the problem.

For example, when you break a bone, the orthopedic surgeon sets the bone, but your body heals the fracture. When you have a bacterial infection, an antibiotic will decrease the number of bacteria in your body, allowing your white blood cells to kill them. These concepts can be applied to healing in general, but it requires a physician willing to listen and take the time to explain.

So, in my opinion, what we need, more than ever, is prevention. We all must be *accountable* for our health and try our hardest to avoid the need for acute medical care. If you can find a patient-focused doctor who listens, that would be ideal.

• • •

If nothing changes, nothing changes.

• • •

As an integrative medicine physician, I see myself as a partner, advocate, and facilitator. Only the patient can choose to change. And, as I have said before if nothing changes, nothing changes. I have seen remarkable changes in patients in my practice. I would guess that at least seventy-five percent are better than before we worked together.

There is nothing more gratifying than for people to NOT need me anymore. The heartbreak comes when those who refuse to change stay the same or get worse. One patient had rheumatoid arthritis (RA). She was looking for miracle cures beyond the medications her rheumatologist gave her—but she ignored the healthy choices right in front of her eyes. She drank five Cokes a day and ate fast food because she was too tired to cook and grocery shop. When I suggested she change these habits, she could not fathom it. She just couldn't go there. She has continued to deteriorate.

On the flip side, I have another RA patient. It took her about a year to change her eating habits, but she stayed consistent with her healthier practices. She lost thirty pounds, and on her last rheumatology visit, she no longer needed the medication. She appears to be in remission. Go figure!

Once you find your partner in healthcare, there are ways you can optimize your relationship as a patient. Here are some of my pearls of wisdom about how to do just that!

Be Organized

Most doctors will only privately admit that they freak out when patients bring in a list of medical complaints. I welcome it. I appreciate when patients can organize their thoughts before coming to see me. It makes my job much easier—just keep the list to one page, please. AskMD will help you record your symptoms in order of importance and give your doctor an excellent printout, along with likely causes. You can access the site online or through their phone app.

Be Open

If you seek out a doctor for their opinion and ideas about improving your health, you will need to leave your own theories and preconceived notions at the door. Many people come in with beliefs that have absolutely no scientific basis. Yet they refuse to listen to reason.

One woman thought the bacteria in her colon were dangerous to her body and wanted me and her gastroenterologist to wipe them all out. That would be impossible, and it would kill her since we need bacteria to live (as you will see when we discuss the gut).

Another patient was profoundly hypothyroid and hypertensive but convinced that dandelion root and iodine were the answers to her problems. She came to me, so I would confirm that. I disagreed and told her she needed medication to control her thyroid and blood pressure. She never returned and died from not properly treating her condition.

Being a partner in wellness means *truly hearing* what your doctor has to say.

Be Honest

Tell your doctor about your symptoms, concerns, and fears.

Many years before I started my integrative medicine practice, I saw a young man in urgent care, who wanted opioid medications for limb pain. I started questioning him and found out what was really going on: his wife was leaving him, and he was devastated. I did not give him the pain medication; I gave him a referral to a therapist.

Many years later, after I started my practice, I saw him at a Relay for Life event. He thanked me and told me that the night he came to see me in urgent care, he had planned to kill himself, and he was going to do it with the pain medication. He took my advice and got help. He told me his life had turned around, and then he introduced me to his lovely new wife and their beautiful baby.

Be Ready to Change

I can give you all the advice in the world, but nothing will change if you are unwilling to change. We know at least eighty percent of disease is due to unhealthy lifestyle choices. If you are willing to improve yours, you will increase your chances of healing. If not, you won't. This straightforward concept is so incredibly hard for most of us to grasp.

I have spent years going through the same drill regarding healthy eating and exercise with a patient I have cared for over the last decade. She suffered from arthritis pain in her knees and back and was always mildly depressed. One day, she decided to follow the lifestyle changes we had discussed. (It took about five years for the concept to sink in.) Once she changed her eating and exercise habits, she lost weight, her knees improved, and so did her mood. For her, it was nothing short of a miracle. Sometimes it takes a while for the message to get through. I am so glad it did for her, and I keep hoping it will work for others, especially after reading this book. The body is a beautiful thing, and this book offers some wonderful doable ideas that are fun and delicious and can lead you on a healing journey.

In the chapters to come…

You will learn about your amazing brain, how it works and why it is crucial to treat it well. The mechanics and possibilities of what it can do will amaze, delight and inspire you to do everything you can to keep it in tip-top shape! (I couldn't resist the pun.)

You will find out what makes your heart tick and why you need it to perform at its best. You will realize how essential it is for your body's other functions. Keeping your heart healthy and well is not a complicated process, but it can be challenging. It requires eating healthy and exercising, which often requires effort and a lifestyle change.

You will learn all about your gut and dive into the world of the microbiome. *Who knew poop could be so fascinating?* That is where you will find all the organisms that make up the gut microbiome. Keeping these microbes healthy and happy will allow you to have a happy, disease-free life. Again, it isn't necessarily complicated, but it can be difficult for people to shift their diet and exercise preferences.

• • •

Who knew poop could be so fascinating?

• • •

And there is so much more on how you can boost your brain, live a long and healthy life, improve your mood, prevent chronic diseases, find balance, and enjoy great sex and sleep. You will learn how to eat healthfully, exercise, and deal with stress in unique and fun ways.

Fortunately, I will give you the tools for better health and teach you why you will want to use them. As I said earlier, the changes outlined in this book are simple but not easy. It can feel uncomfortable or scary, but the reward is worth ten times the effort. I want you to know how these pieces all fit together, what you can do, and most of all, I want you to understand why it's worth it.

It is an honor and pleasure to guide you on an incredible journey to health and wellness. The world was very different when *Healed* was published in 2017. The book was very different too. At that time, the emphasis was on exercise's health benefits, specifically ballroom dance. It is hard to believe what has happened in just five years, but our new reality requires a much more expansive and global view of our lives and health. In *Heal Now* you will find a roadmap you can use to be your best partner in health. It will start at the top of the body and work its way down. To begin with, I want to introduce you to your most fascinating organ, your command center, and your potential for greatness: YOUR BRAIN!

PART ONE

SMARTS, HEARTS, AND FARTS!
THE INTEGRATION OF THE
BRAIN, HEART, AND GUT

D o you ever wonder what would happen If your body organs could talk to each other? Well, believe it or not, they actually can and do! Not only do they communicate, but they integrate. They are intertwined and interdependent. When it comes to the brain, heart, and gut, by affecting one, you affect them all—for better or worse.

The Brain and the Gut

As an example of how the gut affects the brain, a study of 7,000 people found that those who were fed a healthier diet from an early age had higher IQs than those who were not. Children who were breastfed and then had a diet rich in fruits, veggies, and healthy foods also had higher IQs by age 8 when compared to those with unhealthy diets.[1] A healthy diet creates a diverse and balanced microbiome (the microorganisms that inhabit the gut). This is responsible for the positive effects on the brain. There is a positive feedback loop to the brain via the enteric nervous system in the gut that connects to the brain via the vagus nerve. You will learn all about this in The BRAIN 101 and The GUT 101 (pages 3 and 63).

The Gut and the Heart

These same microbes influence the heart. Certain types of gut bacteria are associated with high blood pressure and lower HDL levels or "good" cholesterol.[2]

The TMAO (Trimethylamine N-oxide) story I share in the sections to come is probably one of the best examples. This is a substance made by gut bacteria when red meat, farm-raised fish, and egg yolks (to name a few) are consumed. Elevated levels of TMAO have been associated with increases in the incidence of stroke and heart attack and are proving to correlate better with these outcomes than cholesterol levels. These levels affect both the brain and the heart.[3]

You can see tremendous benefits by simply reducing consumption of these products, eating a whole food plant-based diet, and focusing on healthy lifestyle choices. Just by making even small changes, the payoff is substantial.

The gut and heart communicate through the enteric and autonomic nervous systems. The vagus nerve, called the wandering nerve for good reason because it goes everywhere, is also integral to communication with the heart. You will learn about this in HEART 101.

What About the Heart and the Brain?

When it comes to the heart and brain, you have seen this movie before. Just think about when something has scared or upset you. What happened? Your heart sped up, and your blood pressure probably increased as well. The brain was telling your body to get ready to fight or flee. Part of that transmission could speed up your heart and help you take off if you needed to. It is a complicated chain of events commanded by the brain and communicated to various organs in the body.

Keeping all these systems in tip-top condition is essential. It will maximize your health. If one fails, they are all affected. If one heals, you get bonus points, and they all get better. Understanding the intricacy of these systems and how they relate to each other is essential, and once you do, you will be inspired to keep them healthy. I will start at the top and work my way down.

CHAPTER 1

THE BRAIN

– BRAIN 101–

Your DNA is 99.9% identical to other humans and chimps. Most surprisingly it is 90% identical to every mammal on this planet including dogs, cats, and even elephants! What distinguishes people from each other (and from their pets) are a few differences that, in the scheme of things, are minute. One of the main things that makes you the unique individual you are is your personality and the seat where it resides. That place is your brain. For this reason and more, most scientists agree that the brain is the most important organ in the body. It's command central, responsible for coordinating our actions and reactions and allowing us to think, feel, and remember those thoughts and feelings. Your body can live without the brain (with the help of life support machines), but what's the point?

The brain is where all our senses stem: the enjoyment you get from eating chocolate, smelling the daphne flowers in the spring, hearing Beethoven's Fifth Symphony (or the Seventh, my personal favorite) or a baby's giggle, seeing the gorgeous color and details in artwork or scenery, and feeling the touch and hug of someone you love.

Our minds and imaginations—our ability to solve problems, laugh at a joke, daydream, create, design, build, write, learn something new, enjoy a hobby, and master a skill—are housed and electrified by our brains.

Our brain moves our body. It enables us to tap our toes, walk, dance, leap tall buildings in a single bound (just kidding), shape words in our mouths, use our hands to express our emotions, and run and play with our kids. Everything that makes our lives great, and makes us who we are, is centered in our brain. When our brain's health diminishes, so does our essence. Saving your brain means saving yourself.

Your Remarkable Brain

The brain is remarkable! In addition to all that other great stuff, did you know your brain's storage capacity is considered *virtually unlimited*? Research suggests the human brain consists of about *86 billion neurons*. Each neuron forms connections to other neurons, which could add *up to one quadrillion (1,000 trillion) connections*. Despite the myth that we only use ten percent of our brain, we use most of it. Here are more very cool (actually "hot") facts about the brain.[4]

• • •

The human brain is the only object
that can contemplate itself.

• • •

- **It is HOT.** The brain runs on enough electricity to power a 25-watt bulb. It is the hottest part of the body, set at around 38.5° Celsius (101.3° Fahrenheit). It is much warmer than the core body temperature.[5]

- **It's the Great Connector.** A quadrillion neuronal connections combine and increase storage capacity. These connections are incredibly fast, transmitted at 268 miles an hour. And though the brain is fully formed at age 25, its ability to create new connections remains throughout our lives.[6]

- **And the Thinker.** The human brain is the only object that can contemplate itself. Think about that!

- **It's Pain-Free.** The brain has zero pain receptors. Migraines occur in the lining or meninges covering the brain. Surgeons doing brain surgery often allow the patient to be awake. It is fascinating to watch. The patient does not experience pain. They do this so the patient can tell the surgeon what is happening. When they touch certain areas of the brain, they can avoid damaging essential parts, such as those segments that generate speech and various senses.[7]

• • •

A healthy brain can heal.

• • •

When you realize all the mind-boggling things the brain does, you see how imperative it is to keep it tuned and in good shape. Here are two more reasons: a healthy brain can heal, and a healthy brain can prevent diseases that destroy your quality of life. And conversely, a healthy brain can further enrich the life you're leading. Think of all the fantastic things you can do with it. Your opportunities are limitless when you protect and promote your brain's health. And if unpredictable things happen, at least you will have some brain-power on reserve.

As an example, one of my patients, Fiona, had a significant stroke and was given clot-busting medications. At 62 years old, she recovered to some degree but was still left with right arm and right leg weakness and some slurring of her speech. She was determined to get back to her normal level of function. She worked with physical and speech therapists, and gradually, over about a year, she got almost everything back.

The lack of blood supply caused a part of Fiona's brain to become damaged and some brain cells to die. The healthy area of her brain learned to take over. In this way, she could create new networks and electrical connections. This is called neuroplasticity.

While in the hospital, she started intense strength training with simple activities that had suddenly become very difficult for her, such as squeezing rubber balls. She had to relearn daily living activities, like using a knife and fork and peeling an orange. For speech therapy, she worked on forming words and sentences.

Working with her pet Labrador retriever accelerated her movement and walking. The dog was an excellent motivator for getting her up and out every day once she was discharged from the hospital. Fiona still has a slight limp but has reclaimed the quality of life she had before the stroke. Observing the magnificence of the brain as it heals itself over time is incredible.

And remarkably, when multiple areas are involved, such as learning and enjoying music, memories can be retained regardless of deterioration, like in Alzheimer's disease. In 2021, Tony Bennett was seen singing with Lady Gaga. He has advanced Alzheimer's but was able to remember the song set and performed beautifully. Afterward, Bennett became confused and didn't remember where he was.[8]

From all we know, it is clear that your brain is a miraculous organ. When you think about its capabilities, how it can repair itself in certain circumstances, how it grows in so many ways, and how it makes YOU who you are…it is truly *mind-blowing*. A healthy brain makes our lives what they are: full and rich and interesting.

And it keeps our lives interesting when we never stop learning.

What About Your IQ? Can That Be Increased? Maybe!

Our ability to grow through learning never stops. It may slow down, but it is never too late. Although learning may not be as easy as when we were children, regardless of how old a person is, they can still learn. A study published in 2013 found that senior citizens who acquired a new skill had improved memory. The researchers asked 221 people between the ages of 60 and 90 to take up a new hobby devoting 16.5 hours a week for three months to learning it. One control group did social activities like watching movies. The most significant memory gains were from the learning group. Regardless of their age, they were able to learn a new skill.[9]

A fascinating case study was done in 2005 by Dr. Siegfried Othmer with identical 8-year-old twins who had mild developmental delays and were taught a form of deep meditation that I will explain later in the book. This special form of meditation uses[10] neurofeedback to help boost cognition. After following the meditation protocol, both twins increased their individual IQs by 23 points. Deep meditation slowed the brainwave activity and increased the ability of the brain to reorganize itself![11]

So, you can see why it is so important to keep our brains healthy. This way, even if something unforeseen happens, we have a better chance of repairing it fully. In addition, if we keep it in top shape (so to speak), we can prevent various diseases. There are ways to do that. But first, it's time for a little BRAIN 101.

• • •

Are you a fathead?

• • •

Are You a Fathead? (Yes)

The brain is a relatively complex structure composed of three main parts: the cerebrum, cerebellum, and brainstem. The cerebrum is the largest part of the brain and has right and left hemispheres which communicate with each other through a middle connector, the corpus callosum. The brain weighs about three pounds in an average adult, and 40% consists of water, protein, carbohydrates, and salts. The majority, or 60%, is fat. When I spoke to kids at a local grade school about the brain, I told them if they called their parents fatheads, they would be right! Don't let the joke fool you, though: the brain is a complex network of blood vessels and nerves, with synapses continuously firing. It rests but never fully sleeps. (Interesting aside, when you sleep in a hotel room on a trip, do you notice that you don't feel as rested despite a full night's sleep? That is because half your brain stays awake all night to be on guard in a new environment.)

The Brain is Your Mainframe Computer

The brain runs your body. It controls thought, memory, emotion, touch, motor skills, vision, breathing, temperature, and even hunger. It is in charge of everything that regulates your body. The various parts of the brain oversee different processes. The cerebellum controls balance. The cerebrum controls muscle function, speech, emotion, thought, reading, writing, and learning. The brainstem at the base is the relay center of the brain. It sends information from the brain to the rest of the body. It plays a crucial role in consciousness, awareness, and movement. All the parts of the brain need to be healthy and nourished, and that is where the heart comes in.

The Brain-Heart Connection

The relationship between the brain and the heart is mutually beneficial. The heart provides oxygen via the bloodstream, which keeps the brain nourished. Without the heart providing oxygenated blood to the brain, it would either die or, if circulation is eventually restored (depending on how long it took), it would be damaged.

On the other hand, the brain controls the heart through the brainstem. It does this directly through the sympathetic and parasympathetic branches of the autonomic nervous system. The autonomic nervous system is responsible for the control of bodily functions that are not consciously directed. This includes breathing, heartbeat and digestion.

Sympathetic nerves kick into gear in "fight or flight" mode, causing your heart rate to increase. Parasympathetic nerves keep the heart calm and lower the pulse rate. They are part of an intricate system and work together to balance each other out. Our body works best when this balance happens. Heart rate variability, or HRV, expresses the interplay between the two systems. A high HRV is the healthiest. It means that your heart and body can be calmed and not constantly stressed with a continually elevated pulse. The vagus nerve (which plays a major role in the gut, as you will see) is part of the parasympathetic nervous system and plays a central role in slowing the heart. Keeping both systems in check is vital; otherwise, bad things can happen.

A great example is vasovagal syncope or fainting. Have you seen someone faint at the sight of blood or after witnessing trauma? That is the vagus nerve at work. It causes a sudden drop in heart rate and blood pressure when triggered by certain events. When there is a substantial sympathetic outpouring from trauma or a major stressful event that goes unchecked, the heart can be injured by the massive release of adrenaline. This is called "Broken Heart Syndrome." *All* of this is commandeered by the brain!

The Brain-Gut Connection

The brain-gut connection is one of my favorite topics, and we will be thoroughly discussing it in GUT 101. For now, you need to know that the brain is in direct communication with the gut as well as the heart. Once again, the vagus nerve plays a huge role in connecting the gut's enteric nervous system to the brain. Chemical connections via neurotransmitters, like serotonin, are responsible for the feelings and emotions produced by the brain.[12] Many of these neurotransmitters are made in the brain AND the gut by the microbiome, a collection of microbes that are the multitaskers of the gut. In other words, our gut feels emotions, too. If you get diarrhea when you're nervous, now you know why that happens.

The brain and the body are finely tuned machines. There are controls to keep it balanced, nourished, and healthy. Sometimes things get screwed up beyond our control, such as trauma and accidents. However, most things are within our control, and there are ways to prevent dreaded diseases. Granted, some people may have a genetic predisposition toward Alzheimer's disease and Parkinson's; however, that does not mean you are doomed to have them, only that your chances are greater than those without a genetic predisposition. If you take charge of your health and wellness, you can avoid them.

Alzheimer's disease, Parkinson's disease, and Traumatic Brain Injury (TBI) can be improved, delayed, and possibly prevented by proper nutrition, specific measures, and particular types of activity. Strokes are included in the discussion of the heart.

Alzheimer's Disease

Whenever I ask patients what their biggest fear is regarding their health, the answer is unanimous. They are most afraid of losing their minds. If you gave people a choice between getting cancer or Alzheimer's, the vast majority would pick cancer.

According to the Alzheimer's Association as of 2022, more than five and a half million Americans were living with Alzheimer's disease. Every 67 seconds another person begins developing this form of dementia. It is estimated that 500,000 people die because of the disease every year. However, that number is falsely low. The statistic is taken from death certificates and while many patients may have Alzheimer's disease leading to various events that result in death (such as a fractured hip, a head injury, or an infection), the condition is not listed as the cause of death. The immediate cause of death is what is placed on the death certificate; most commonly, cardiac or respiratory failure.[13]

These statistics may lead you to believe that Alzheimer's disease is on the rise. However, over the years the incidences of Alzheimer's and dementia, in general, have actually been decreasing. A 2001 study found that from 1993 to 1998, it decreased from

6.1% to 3.8%. And, over the last 30 years, dementia has declined by around 13% every decade for those of European ancestry living in the US. What *has* increased is the number of people living into their 60s and beyond. That is why it looks like dementia is on the rise, when in truth, it is the population prone to dementia that is on the rise.[14]

Alzheimer's is a progressive brain disease that destroys memory and thinking skills. It generally appears in the mid-60s age group and beyond but can occur earlier. It is the most common cause of dementia in the elderly. However, it was rare when first discovered and diagnosed in 1906 when Dr. Alois Alzheimer noticed changes in the brain tissue of a 55-year-old woman named Auguste D., who had died of an unusual mental illness. At age 50, Auguste D. was described as having memory loss, language problems, and unpredictable behavior. After she died, Dr. Alzheimer examined her brain and found abnormal clumps or plaques of a material we now call amyloid. There were tangled bundles of fibers as well, which are now considered the main pathologic feature of the disease. Unfortunately, Alzheimer's colleagues showed little interest in his findings.[15]

However, a fellow physician did diagnose a male patient, Josef F., with Alzheimer's disease before the patient died. The patient lived three years with the disease before passing away at age 51. An autopsy showed the plaque *without* the tangles, indicating the disease may not have been as advanced as in the patient seen by Dr. Alzheimer, or it was a variation of the disease. It wasn't until 1995, when the slides from Josef F. and others were intensively reviewed, that Dr. Alzheimer was credited with showing the progression of the disease in different stages. You might wonder why others in the early 1900s did not jump on board and readily acknowledge the condition. One of the reasons may be that it was not prevalent. In 1900, the average life expectancy was 47 years of age. Since Alzheimer's shows up later in life, relatively few had the disease.[16]

What Are the Signs?

Joanne was an 82-year-old woman who had been a brilliant, successful dynamo most of her life. She lived in a major city with a demanding, fast-paced job which she performed efficiently and enthusiastically. In her late seventies, things started to shift. She started forgetting things. It started with names and directions. Then her personality started to change. She became paranoid and felt as if she was being watched. She began hiding things around the house. When she went to restaurants, she tried to sneak silverware into her purse. She would forget she had eaten dinner and try to order another meal. The small drops of spilled chocolate ice cream on her shirt—she loved chocolate ice cream after dinner—was the only way to prove that she had already eaten.

As time went on, Joanne became more of a recluse. Her body remained healthy as her mind started slipping away. She became very childlike. At first, she gained weight because she was eating multiple meals. However, she gradually forgot how to eat and swallow and became very thin. Finally, she forgot how to drink water, and she died.

To the very end, there were tiny moments of recognition that gave a fleeting glimpse of the person Joanne used to be, and then the person she had become would be back. It was so hard for everyone around her to watch her progression. It was hard for me as well. Joanne was my mother-in-law.

We saw signs of Joanne's dementia that progressed over years. Often the early signs are subtle and likely to be noticed only by those close to the person. Here are a few things to look for.

Personality Change

The first thing I have noticed in my patients who have developed Alzheimer's disease is the loss of their sense of humor. A patient of mine from many years ago named Jan was one of my favorite patients because she was so fun and bubbly. Jan was a Japanese woman who married a serviceman and moved to Oregon. She raised a family and looked forward to traveling after her husband retired. I cared for her for seven years before she and her husband retired and left the area. Roughly ten years later, her husband brought Jan to see me. She was no longer the fun-loving, jovial person I remembered. Furthermore, she did not know who I was. It was alarming, to say the least.

In addition to losing her sense of humor, Jan developed paranoia and delusions, also common in the disease. She repeatedly called the police because she thought her husband was holding her captive. She would lock herself in the bathroom to hide and feel safe. Jan was diagnosed with advanced Alzheimer's disease; sadly, she died about a year later.

Disordered Thinking

Loss of short-term memory is another early sign. Patients commonly forget appointments, words, and names. They will often have sticky notes all over as memory aids.

Trouble with Visual and Spatial Images

As the disease progresses, perception may change. Patients misjudge distances and angles. Hopefully, they will stop driving because they will have great difficulty and soon become dangerous behind the wheel.

Patients may not recognize their reflection in the mirror, leading to or increasing their paranoia. They also may have trouble distinguishing colors. One of the tests used to diagnose the disease is asking patients to draw a clock and put in a specific time. Patients with Alzheimer's typically cannot visualize the clock and cannot place the numbers and minute and hour hands in the appropriate place.

Trouble Planning and Tracking

One of the first things to go is the ability to keep a checkbook. (Frankly, I gave up trying to balance my checkbook in the 1980s, so that test doesn't count for those of us who have embraced online banking and debit cards.) Performing other simple tasks may become difficult. For example, using the remote for the TV or setting a microwave may become impossible. (Again, that would be for those who could do it in the first place.)

Confusion About the Time and Date

Disorientation regarding time and date is a common symptom of Alzheimer's. Almost everyone tends to forget what day it is when on vacation. However, forgetting is not normal when you are in your weekly/monthly routine. Many patients will be unclear regarding the date, time of year, or time of day.

Difficulty Finding the Correct Word

We all forget names and sometimes lose words from time to time. Alzheimer's patients lose words frequently. They often have trouble maintaining and/or following a conversation. One of my patients was quite eloquent and loved to talk. I knew something was up when she rarely would converse, and when we did talk, she would get confused and agitated.

Misplacing Things and Putting Them in Unusual Places

One of my patients would take things and put them in odd places. Like my mother-in-law, she developed an affinity for silverware. She often tried to take forks and spoons from restaurants and put them in her purse. At home, her husband found silverware all over the house: under mattresses, in the freezer, and in the laundry room. She put the house keys in the refrigerator and the remote control in the pantry. It is normal to forget where you put things. Putting them in strange places is a sign something may be wrong.

Poor Judgment

Patients with Alzheimer's may start to make poor decisions, particularly regarding money. They are easy prey for telemarketers and scam artists because they lose the ability to discern what is legit and what is not.

One of my patients gave the majority of her money away to her college alumni association. It was very nice of her, and the college appreciated her, but she left nothing for her children.

How Is Alzheimer's Disease Diagnosed?

The only way to definitively diagnose Alzheimer's is at autopsy. Many tests can lead to the diagnosis, but no test can tell with 100% certainty that a patient has the disease. The main tests are:

Neuropsychiatric Testing

When family members and patients start to notice changes, as we mentioned above, most doctors first order neuropsychiatric testing. Psychologists evaluate cognitive function, allowing them to diagnose possible decline. These tests include problem-solving, memory, attention, counting, and language skills. They can distinguish dementia from other problems, such as depression and emotional disorders.

Medical Tests

Blood and urine tests can help rule out other causes of memory loss. Thyroid disease, vitamin deficiencies, and certain infectious diseases such as Lyme disease and syphilis can mimic this form of dementia.

Brain Scans

Brain scans such as computed tomography (CT) and magnetic resonance imaging (MRI), and positron emission tomography (PET) are pretty helpful. The CT and MRI scans can show other possible causes of dementia, such as stroke and infection. They can also show the loss or shrinkage of brain tissue. There is quite a bit of excitement surrounding the use of PET scans because they can show amyloid deposits in the brain. These are suggestive but not conclusively diagnostic for Alzheimer's disease, as some people have evidence of plaques but no disease.

What Are the Treatments?

There are medications that help slow the progression of the disease. These include Aricept and Namenda. While there is currently no drug that reverses or stops the ravages of Alzheimer's, some promising new treatments are being studied.[17]

Let's first talk about some treatment basics.

Food for Thought (Literally!)

A well-balanced diet may make a difference in keeping our brains healthy. Studies have found that diets rich in green leafy vegetables and cruciferous vegetables such as broccoli and Brussels sprouts maintain healthy brain function.

Several studies have confirmed that when people followed the Mediterranean diet, they had a lower risk of developing Alzheimer's. One study in particular saw a 28% lower risk of developing the very early stage of the disease, called mild cognitive impairment. Those who maintained the diet had a 48% lower chance of progressing from mild cognitive impairment to full-blown Alzheimer's.[17] This diet is rich in whole foods, including vegetables, fruits, legumes, whole grains, lean protein, olive oil, and the occasional glass of red wine.

Fish Oil May Be Another Effective Tool for Prevention

Fish oil has been found to help the memory of mice bred to have Alzheimer's. The mice develop amyloid plaque in their brains. These plaques are suspected of being part of the cause of Alzheimer's in humans. Mice given a diet rich in omega-3 fatty acids had fewer plaque deposits than those not given fish oil.[18] Unfortunately, the same results have not been seen in people. It has been suggested supplementation with fish oil needs to be started early before the cognitive decline starts happening.

New Medical Therapies?

One of the other possible causes of this disease is that the brain becomes resistant to insulin. In theory, a diabetes medication called Metformin might halt and possibly reverse cognitive impairment. In fact, a study in 2020 found patients with diabetes and cognitive dysfunction showed marked cognitive improvement after taking Metformin.[19]

A study using the mice mentioned above has found the diabetes drug Victoza (Liraglutide) was able to expedite the removal of the amyloid plaque from the brains of the mice with Alzheimer's and return to their normal cognitive function. This drug is injected daily and lowers blood sugar without causing hypoglycemia or low blood sugar. The drug is currently being studied in Alzheimer's patients and is showing some promise.[20]

A small study done in Canada has found Alzheimer's patients treated with intravenous immunoglobulin showed no further cognitive decline after three treatments. Researchers believe the antibodies in the immunoglobulin halted the inflammation that causes beta-amyloid to be formed in the brain. Further clinical trials on this promising treatment are ongoing.[21]

In 2016, researchers reported inspiring results of a small study called the metabolic enhancement for neurodegeneration, or MEND program, conducted with nine patients who had early Alzheimer's disease and one with advanced disease. Recognizing that single or monotherapies have been unsuccessful in reversing Alzheimer's, they decided to try a multi-pronged approach personalized for each patient.[17]

For example, one female patient eliminated all simple carbohydrates from her diet, resulting in a twenty-pound weight loss. She eliminated all gluten and processed foods, increasing her intake of fruit, vegetables, and wild fish. She reduced stress with yoga and meditation 20 minutes twice a day. She took melatonin (0.5 mg) at bedtime, vitamin D (2000 IU daily), and CoQ10 (200 mg daily). She started flossing regularly and used an electric toothbrush. She had stopped her hormones years before fearing the risk of breast cancer after a correlation between hormone replacement therapy and breast cancer was hyped in the media. However, assessing that she had no increased risk for breast cancer and that the benefit from taking hormone replacement was substantial, the MEND program doctors suggested she resume taking her hormone replacement therapy. She fasted twelve hours between dinner and breakfast and exercised at least thirty minutes four to five days a week. Two and a half years after entering the study, her symptoms reversed, and she remains asymptomatic.

Others with high cholesterol were treated to optimize their levels with diet and medication. Those who needed vitamin B12 were supplemented, and others were given minerals such as copper and zinc. Although these changes were difficult for patients to follow, the results kept them in the program, and nine out of ten have maintained their improvements. More extensive trials will be forthcoming.

• • •

New on the horizon

• • •

What Is New on the Horizon?

Since 2021, scientists at MIT seem to be making "headway" when treating Alzheimer's disease utilizing electrical pulses called gamma waves in the brain. The researchers noticed that these waves become weaker and less synchronized in people with Alzheimer's. They thought they might be able to slow down the disease by boosting gamma waves. First studied in mice, they found that mice exposed to certain lights and sounds caused the gamma waves in their brains to strengthen and synchronize. This was very effective in mice bred to have Alzheimer's disease. Their brains cleared out amyloid and tau (tangled) proteins after treatment. Their immune cells functioned better, and the mice improved on tests for memory and learning.[22]

But what about humans? The research team built a portable device to generate light and sound pulses at the correct frequency (40 Hz). They sent it home with patients with mild Alzheimer's dementia. They had them use it for an hour every day for three months. The patients were then checked for atrophy or brain loss.

Those who used the device had no atrophy over that time. Those given a placebo device did. The small study was only done on 15 people, with a larger study in the works, but this treatment could be a real game changer.[23]

Another Possible Game Changer

Transcranial magnetic stimulation, or TMS, is another promising treatment presently used in the treatment of depression. It utilizes noninvasive stimulation techniques and passes electrical impulses through a small coil of wire on the scalp. This generates a magnetic field that passes into the brain past the skull while the device rests on the surface. Scientists have found that placing the impulses over the brain's prefrontal cortex greatly improved depression. By utilizing other areas during experimentation, memory improves in healthy people. Small trials have found improvement in cognition in Alzheimer's patients. More extensive trials to look at safety and enhance brain function are planned.[24]

One More Possibility

When it comes to the brain, the first line of defense against invaders is immune cells, which vacuum up amyloid and toxic substances. As we age, these cells weaken and aren't as prone to picking up the vacuum. Amyloid found in Alzheimer's disease may accumulate because of this. Researchers at MIT are focusing on these cells. If the immune cells can be energized, they might slow or even prevent the process of Alzheimer's. This is another promising approach. Lecanemab, a new drug released in 2023 utilizes this mechanism and has shown promise.[25]

What You Can Do Now to Say Adios to Alzheimer's Disease!

We have established that no treatments are available to halt or reverse Alzheimer's (yet), so we must find ways to prevent it. There appear to be a few things that may have an impact: healthy eating, social engagement, and exercise.

Alfred is a 72-year-old gentleman who lived alone after losing his wife to ovarian cancer. His family was worried when he started to lose his way home. Their concern was intensified because he had a strong family history of Alzheimer's disease. To soothe his loneliness, Alfred took up ballroom dancing, and things changed dramatically. Soon after he started dance classes, his thinking became clear, and he was much happier. Alfred met a lovely woman at his favorite dance venue, and the two started dancing together several times a week. He and his dancing friend have continued for over ten years. Alfred's mental function has remained intact; he has never developed any signs of dementia, and neither has his partner, who is well into her 90s.

Exercise is essential, and when it comes to Alzheimer's, so is social engagement. One of the most fascinating studies to date on this subject is the Nun Study, a longitudinal study started in 1986 following over 700 nuns and priests, observing their mental and physical health throughout their lives—and beyond. Their activities, thoughts, and feelings are monitored, noted, and cataloged. They have yearly physical and cognitive exams. They have donated their bodies to science, and their brains are analyzed when they die.

Now well beyond its 30th year, the study has found those who frequently participated in activities such as listening to the radio, reading newspapers, playing puzzle games, and visiting museums were 47% less likely to develop Alzheimer's than those who did not. What is most intriguing about this study is that fifteen nuns showed *no* signs of dementia in life, but when their brains were analyzed, they were diagnosed with severe Alzheimer's. Their brains were loaded with the telltale plaque associated with the disease. The researchers wondered how that could be possible. On a pathologic exam, they had Alzheimer's but in life, they did not!

So, they looked back at their writing and activities and found those women had a strong positive outlook and a sense of purpose. Being active is also essential, and finding an activity encouraging social engagement is a win-win.[26]

Exercise is vital for general health. A healthy heart and vascular system are essential for a healthy brain. The question is, which activities provide the *most* benefit? As I mentioned in the Prologue, in 2003 a study published in the *New England Journal of Medicine* helped answer that question. Researchers studied 469 people between the ages of 75 and 85. Participants responded to surveys that addressed their activities, such as walking, bicycling, reading, doing crossword puzzles, and dancing. They were followed for five years. At the end of the study, 124 had dementia.

Those who danced frequently had a lower risk of dementia when compared to those who did not. The risk of dementia was reduced by 0% in those who were regular cyclists and swimmers, 0% for regular golfers, 35% reduced in those who were regular readers, 47% reduced by those who did crossword puzzles at least four times a week—and lowered by a stunning 76% for those who were partner dancing two to three times a week.[27]

Scientists have studied why dancing is so good for the brain. The cerebral cortex and the hippocampus parts of the brain are very plastic and can be easily rewired. That is a good thing. The downside is if you don't use them, you lose them. Partner dancing requires multiple split-second decisions that are great for exercising the brain, therefore keeping these essential parts of the brain highly functional.[28] As we age, creating more neural pathways in the brain improves brain function and gives us more reserve in the event that there is an injury, and in the meantime, it keeps us mentally sharp.

One might look at the study above and wonder about the results since the activities were self-reported and were observational rather than a proper clinical trial. You might ask the question: has a clinical trial ever looked at subjects before and after dance training? And the answer is, *Yes*. The researchers looked at dancing the Cha-Cha and cognitive function in older subjects. Thirty-eight seniors with metabolic syndrome (prediabetes) with normal cognitive function were divided into two groups. One group danced the Cha-Cha twice a week for six months, and the other group followed their regular exercise routine. The dancing group showed improved cognition compared to the other control group. The researchers concluded this by looking at verbal fluency, word list recall, and recognition after a time delay.

What effect is seen in the brain with this type of activity? Radiologists at the University of California Los Angeles were able to shed some light on this.[29] They studied 20 years of data from a group of 876 adults who averaged 78 years of age. This data looked at weight and height, and lifestyle habits. They used special scans using magnetic resonance imaging (MRI) that established 3D images of the brains of these individuals. With these, they could measure the amount of gray matter in the brain used for memory and decision-making. The more gray matter, the more brain power—and this area shrinks in those with Alzheimer's disease. The researchers found that those who were the most active had more gray matter than those who were not. A combination of healthy lifestyle choices and activities was most beneficial. The researchers attributed these positive changes to improved blood flow to the brain and stronger neural connections.[30]

The bottom line is that to keep from losing brain function, we need to harness our brainpower. Embracing a healthy lifestyle with a whole-food, Mediterranean-style diet, social interaction, and exercise can do it. However, not just any activity will do when it comes to growing neural connections and protecting the brain from Alzheimer's. Crossword puzzles and reading can help with brain exercise. However, ballroom dancing is the best choice for the most beneficial and expeditious results. It exercises the body as well as the mind and is fun. It also provides many other benefits, as you will soon see.

Parkinson's Disease

Another disease that strikes fear into people's hearts and has no cure is Parkinson's, a degenerative nervous system disorder; a chronic and progressive condition. It can take a while for people to receive a diagnosis. Here is a story from one of my patients.

Theresa is a 65-year-old woman who has always been active. She noticed she was developing a tremor and her balance was off. Theresa would feel as if she were falling forward when she walked. Sometimes she would just freeze and not be able to keep going. Her family noticed she no longer smiled, and her voice was also shaky. She complained of pain and stiffness in her arms. She went to her doctor, who suspected she had Parkinson's disease, and the neurologist she was referred to confirmed the diagnosis. She was treated with medications and was able to regain some of her movements. Ultimately, she was given a revolutionary device; a pacemaker for the brain. Known as deep brain stimulation, the pacemaker device is implanted in a special portion of the brain. When stimulated it reduces symptoms such as tremors, and rigidity. This has transformed her life by allowing her to have hours during the day when she is moving in a relatively normal way. More on this later.[31]

What Are the Symptoms?

There are four main symptoms of Parkinson's disease:

Tremor

The classic tremor in Parkinson's disease is a rhythmic back-and-forth motion that involves the thumb and forefinger and is described as pill rolling. It is most apparent at rest, disappears during sleep, and improves with intentional movement.

Rigidity

Rigidity or resistance to movement is a common symptom. The muscles are tense and contracted, so they cause stiffness and pain. It becomes most apparent as someone tries to move a patient's arm. It becomes rigid and resists movement, resulting in a cogwheel motion.

Bradykinesia

Defined as an abnormal slowness of movement, the patient affected cannot perform routine motions quickly. The facial expression will also stiffen.

Loss Of Balance

Parkinson's causes patients to be unstable. They will often fall over, whether standing or sitting, but Parkinson's symptoms usually start on one side of the body. As the disease progresses, it affects both sides. People begin to walk with a gait that causes them to lean forward and take hurried steps. They may have trouble initiating movement and stop suddenly as they walk and then freeze.

Other Symptoms

People have difficulty walking, talking, and completing simple tasks. The disease eventually causes patients to become wheel-chair-bound or even wholly bedridden. They often develop dementia. Swallowing becomes difficult, and they can develop aspiration pneumonia and chronic bronchitis. Forty-four percent of patients die as a result of complications from pneumonia and bronchitis.[32]

Speech is affected in half of the patients, causing them to speak softly and in a monotone. Other accompanying symptoms include urinary difficulty, oily skin and hair, sleeping difficulties, memory problems, and trouble maintaining blood pressure while standing. Fatigue and loss of energy are also quite common, along with emotional changes. It is a life-changing, terribly burdensome disease.

Who Gets It?

It is estimated that 50,000 Americans are diagnosed with Parkinson's every year. It affects 50% more men than women. The usual age of onset is around 60 years. Those with one or more close relatives with the disease are at higher risk. Scientists have identified several genetic mutations associated with Parkinson's disease.[33]

What Causes It?

Parkinson's disease occurs when nerve cells in the brain die or become damaged. The central part of the brain affected is the substantia nigra. The cells in this area produce dopamine. This is a chemical messenger responsible for transmitting signals between the substantia nigra and the corpus striatum, also known as the relay station of the brain, that produces smooth movements. Loss of dopamine causes the abnormal firing of these signals. Studies have found Parkinson's patients have lost 60- 80% or more of their dopamine-producing cells by the time symptoms appear.[34]

Parkinson's is a disease of the entire body. It is believed the disease starts in the peripheral nervous system in an area such as the intestine, where symptoms such as constipation can be present for years before it is diagnosed.

Toxins

There are certain toxins linked to Parkinson's disease. They may cause the disease by altering genes with mutations similar to those related to hereditary Parkinson's disease. Metal manganese and a drug known as MPTP (1-methyl-4- phenyl-1,2,3,6-tetrahydropyridine), an industrial chemical and a contaminant of illicit narcotics, have both been found to cause Parkinson's disease.[35]

Drugs

Certain drugs prescribed for patients with psychiatric problems, such as chlorpromazine and haloperidol, can cause a reversible form of Parkinson's. Medicines, such as one used for stomach problems, metoclopramide, and a seizure medication known as valproate, can also cause a reversible form of the disease.[36]

Other Causes

Damage as a result of multiple strokes can cause a type of Parkinson's disease. Similarly, frequent head injuries, such as that seen in boxers like Muhammad Ali, can also cause the disease. A viral infection may be another potential cause. I would like to share my grandmother's story to give some additional perspective. It has particular relevance when we see that the COVID epidemic is similar to what she experienced.

My grandmother, Toby, was born in 1900 but was definitely not a typical Victorian woman. She was a self-sufficient businesswoman and prided herself on being independent. She traveled all over the world. Later in her life, at age 75, she developed Parkinson's, and there is some evidence as to why. As a teen, she was afflicted by the Spanish flu epidemic in 1918. At that time, a severe flu outbreak killed millions worldwide, including at least 675,000 Americans.[37] She talked about that time when so many people she knew lost their lives; it was frightening for those who had to live through it. Those who did felt lucky to have survived. Unfortunately, these survivors found themselves at higher risk of developing Parkinson's disease directly following the exposure and later in life, suggesting an infectious component to developing the disease.[38] I believe my Grandma Toby was one of those afflicted. Hopefully, this is not a cautionary tale for those who have survived COVID. Only time will tell.

The Microbiome

The microbiome is a system you will be learning a lot about in GUT 101. However, I need to mention it in connection with Parkinson's disease. The microbiome is made up of microbes (bacteria, fungi, and viruses) that are present in the gut. When they are balanced and living nicely together, they keep your body healthy; when they are out of whack, they can wreak havoc. In December 2022, investigators published a paper on how they believe Parkinson's disease occurs. They found an overabundance of pathogens and immune components in the gut connected to inflammation, toxic molecules, and harmful bacteria forming abnormal proteins. Parkinson's is caused by a dysregulation in the neurotransmitter L-dopa, and that dysregulation is what is occurring in the gut with these inflammatory changes. Knowing this, scientists may be able to find a possible treatment and even (fingers crossed) a cure.[39]

Treatments

Currently, there is no cure for Parkinson's disease. Treatment is aimed at reducing symptoms by boosting dopamine levels or keeping it from being broken down and picked up by receptors so more is available to the brain, or by using drugs that mimic dopamine. There are a variety of medications, such as L–Dopa, that can help. There is also a type of brain surgery that has been effective. A pacemaker is placed in the globus pallidus, which is in the basal ganglia. This stimulation improves Parkinson's symptoms. It is a fairly extreme treatment used for those who have failed medications.[33]

How to Stop Shaking, Rattling, and Rolling!

Even if you haven't had direct experience with Parkinson's disease, you may be aware of the condition because of the actor Michael J. Fox. By his choice to stay in the public eye and continue to work while he struggles with the disease, we have all become familiar with what it does.

The story of Carlos is an excellent example of a patient who has the disease and has found a way to manage it. He is a 61-year-old accomplished ballroom dancer who has been dancing Salsa for years. He started noticing hand and arm tremors at age 47 and was diagnosed with Parkinson's disease seven years later. Parkinson's disease makes movement difficult and requires the need to be conscious of every step. For Carlos, walking is a chore. Eight years ago, he started dancing the Argentine tango. He noticed it made his movement easier. He realized Parkinson's disease keeps his weight over his heels, and tango helps to keep his body forward and improves his backward stride and balance.

Tango keeps Carlos moving. Every morning, he watches his favorite tango dancer on YouTube. Inspired by this man, Carlos puts on his tango music and practices his stride. He credits tango and dance with the ability to ride his bike and walk wherever he needs to go. His dance instructor finds that when Carlos dances, his whole body relaxes into the dance, and his tremors decrease.

Carlos's goal is to retire early so he can have more fun and dance more often.

Parkinson's is a progressive disease of the nervous system. In essence, patients have a deficiency of a chemical called dopamine transmitted by the nervous system. As a result, patients develop tremors, rigid muscles, and poor balance with the tendency to fall forward. Some patients experience "freezing," which is the temporary, involuntary inability to move. This increases the likelihood of falling. It can be perilous.

Therapy focuses on exercise and stretching. This is tough for many patients to do consistently. However, there is a form of physical activity that patients *like* to do. This activity is ballroom dancing, more specifically, tango.[40]

An esteemed Parkinson's researcher, Dr. Gammon Earhart, and her team did a study in 2009 at Washington University, St. Louis. They took 52 patients with Parkinson's disease with similar movement and balance problems. Half the group was given tango lessons twice weekly for a year, and the other half maintained their usual activity level. Improvement in symptoms of Parkinson's disease was noted in many of the tango students. They were able to walk faster and farther, and their balance improved. The non-tango group either remained unchanged or worsened over the years. Those who did the tango also were more active in their lives. They became more social, did more daily activities at home, such as gardening and shopping, and enjoyed going to movies and eating out. These improvements diminished when they stopped dancing. However, most people in the study enjoyed doing the tango and continued to dance.[41]

You may ask, why *tango*? These same researchers looked at the effects of other forms of ballroom dancing on movement and balance for Parkinson's disease patients.

In another study, 58 untreated patients with Parkinson's disease were randomly assigned to one of three groups, a control group with no intervention, a Waltz/Foxtrot group, or a Tango group. They had 20 training sessions over 13 weeks.

Both dance groups improved their balance, motor ability, and walking. The control group worsened by 24% on scales that rate the above factors. Tango was superior to Waltz and Foxtrot when it came to freezing movements in Parkinson's disease. In addition, the speed and stride length of walking improved more with tango.[42]

What is it about dance, and specifically tango, that may be helping? First, dancing offers external cues for movement from the music and a partner. These cues bypass the part of the brain that is dysfunctional. This, in turn, improves gait and coordination. A touch from a partner enhances balance. In tango, visual clues that involve stepping over a partner's foot or crossing one foot over another help prevent the severe symptom of Parkinson's, known as freezing of the gait. The need for forward and backward steps in tango is particularly therapeutic for those with Parkinson's disease.

A particular radiologic imaging test called a PET (positron emission tomography) scan shows brain activity in real-time. A PET scan of the tango dancers revealed that when tango movements were done to a regular, predictable beat, it increased activity in the part of the brain that is dysfunctional in Parkinson's patients.[43]

It is challenging for many of us to get motivated to exercise. For Parkinson's disease patients who suffer from muscle pain and rigidity, loss of balance, and generalized stiffness, it is even more challenging. Tango offers pain relief, improvement in balance, and a better quality of life. The best part is it is fun and very inexpensive. All you need is a decent pair of shoes and a tango class.

You also may want to visit the website **danceforparkinsons.org**. It offers extensive information and opportunities to explore dance as a viable therapy for patients with Parkinson's disease.

$$\bullet \ \bullet \ \bullet$$

One more thing about dance

$$\bullet \ \bullet \ \bullet$$

In Israel, there is a famous economist named Rafi Eldor who was diagnosed with Parkinson's disease in 2008. His doctors told him there was nothing he could do to stop the progression. He found a way. He started dancing. He did so well that he became a world-champion cha-cha dancer. He is able to move normally and halt the progression of his disease. Check out his video entitled "Dance Through Life." You will be inspired regardless of whether you or someone you know has Parkinson's disease.[44]

What About Boxing?

You might think this is an odd question considering that boxing and head trauma can cause Parkinson's disease. A type of boxing has been lifesaving to Parkinson's patients. It is called Rock Steady Boxing. Staying flexible and mobile is essential. It is vital for the body but also for the soul. Rock Steady Boxing does this as a no-contact form of boxing that involves stretching, strength training, and agility work, along with work on motor control.

When those with Parkinson's do this regularly, they can build new neural networks, bypassing the damaged brain areas. The progression of the disease slows and, in some people, reverses to some degree.

And for the Voice

Being able to speak and be heard is essential. This becomes difficult for many people with Parkinson's. There is a program to help with that. It is called SPEAK OUT!®. This is a clinically proven speech therapy program for those with Parkinson's. It utilizes education, speech therapy, home practice, group therapy, and regular assess-ments, allowing people to regain and maintain their speaking ability.

For those with Parkinson's disease, there is hope. Some alternative treatments are being studied as well. Fecal transplant has been used in a few patients and reversed the symptoms for up to three months. This is encouraging, and there will be more studies and possibilities.[45]

Traumatic Brain Injury (TBI)

Traumatic brain injury, also known as TBI, has increased in the modern era. It is an acquired brain injury. The National Institutes of Health describes a TBI as when physical, external forces impact the brain from a penetrating object or a bump, blow, or jolt to the head. Not all blows or jolts to the head result in a TBI. For the ones that do, TBI can range from mild (a brief change in mental status or consciousness) to severe (an extended period of unconsciousness or amnesia after the injury).

TBI affects between 2.5 and 6.5 million Americans. Survivors are often left with significant cognitive, behavioral, and communicative disabilities. An excellent example of this is what happened to a former patient.

Here is his story:

John, a 19-year-old competitive dancer, was returning from a dance competition and had car trouble. He pulled his car over to the side of the road to wait for a tow truck. As he was waiting, he took a bite of a sandwich he had packed and, at the same time, was hit by a guy driving and texting at 80 miles per hour. Not only was his seat belt sheared off, but the impact also caused him to aspirate his sandwich and block his trachea. He had a severe cervical spine injury and was comatose for over a week.

When he awakened, he had difficulty walking, talking, and thinking clearly. No one expected him to make a full recovery. He underwent intensive rehabilitation, and with the help of a specific activity (which we will discuss soon), he is back and better than ever.

What Are the Causes?

According to data from the Centers for Disease Control and Prevention (CDC) and the National Institutes of Health, falls are the most common cause of TBI and occur most frequently among the youngest and oldest age groups. From 2006 to 2010, falls caused more than half (55%) of TBIs among children aged 14 and younger.

Among Americans age 65 and older, falls accounted for more than two-thirds (81%) of all reported TBIs.[46]

The second and third most common causes of TBI are unintentional blunt trauma (accidents that involve being struck by or against an object), followed closely by motor vehicle accidents. Blunt trauma is pervasive in children younger than 15, causing nearly a quarter of all TBIs. Assaults account for an additional 10 percent of TBI and include abuse related TBI, such as head injuries that result from the shaken baby syndrome.

Half of TBI incidents in adults involve alcohol. The severity of the outcome is related to the cause. Ninety-one percent of TBIs due to firearms result in death, whereas only 11% of falls result in death.

Types of TBI

Many types of brain injuries vary depending on the severity and type of injury. There are two broad types of head injuries: penetrating and non-penetrating.

Penetrating TBI (also known as *open* TBI) occurs when the skull is pierced by an object (for example, a bullet, shrapnel, bone fragment, or by a weapon such as a hammer, knife, or baseball bat). With this injury, the object enters the brain tissue. Non-penetrating TBI (also known as *closed head injury* or *blunt* TBI) is caused by an external force that produces brain movement within the skull. Causes include falls, motor vehicle crashes, sports injuries, or being struck by an object. Blast injury due to explosions is a focus of intense study, but how it causes brain injury is not fully known.

One of the most common types of injury is concussion *from a non-penetrating injury*. It is a type of mild TBI that may be considered a temporary injury to the brain but could take minutes to several months to heal. A concussion can be caused by many things, including a bump, a blow or a jolt to the head, a sports injury or fall, a motor vehicle accident, a weapons blast, or a rapid acceleration or deceleration of the brain within the skull (such as the person having been violently shaken). Beyond concussion, the injuries can increase in severity depending on the cause ranging from blood clots, severe bruising, and bleeding to skull fractures.[47]

Complications

Depending on the severity of the injury, complications can occur. Seizures, infection, pain, and injuries of the nerves to the face are among them. Twenty-five percent of those with brain contusions or hematomas and 50 percent of patients with penetrating head trauma develop seizures immediately. Headache is the most common symptom of TBI. Even those with a mild injury can suffer post-concussion syndrome.

The symptoms include headaches, dizziness, vertigo, memory problems, trouble concentrating, sleep, restlessness, irritability, apathy, depression, and anxiety. Many patients may have difficulty speaking and writing and may have visual perception problems. These head injuries also increase the risk of Parkinson's disease, Alzheimer's disease, and post-traumatic dementia.[48]

What Can Be Done?

Physical rehabilitation is essential. In addition, speech therapy, occupational therapy, and vision therapy may be required.

Prevention

The best solution to the problem of TBI is to avoid it in the first place. The important thing is to wear a seatbelt when riding in a car and a helmet when riding a bicycle or a motorcycle. I have noticed that many adult bicyclists often choose *not* to wear helmets. I rarely see children without them. I feel many adult riders think they are good enough and that they won't fall. That may be true; however, the other people on the road are the problem. Just as motorcyclists must be careful of those driving cars and other motorcycles, bicyclists are also vulnerable.

Dr. Olga Jonasson was one of our teachers in medical school. She was a renowned surgeon known for pioneering kidney transplants. Illinois did not have a helmet law at the time and still doesn't. She was famous for driving up to motorcyclists not wearing helmets and offering them an organ donor card. I am sure it gave a few of them pause. At least, I hope it did.

Be sure to keep those helmets on when playing football, baseball, rollerblading, or skateboarding. And keep them on for winter sports, too: snowboarding, skiing, ice skating, and hockey (or make sure your organ donor card is up to date).

Finally, keep all guns locked away along with the bullets stored separately. GSI (gunshot injuries, also known as GSW or gunshot wounds) make for the worst TBI of all.

• • •

"Dance is my passion, my motivation, my future."

• • •

TBI: Dance Away the Trauma

There is very little research on the use of dance for traumatic brain injury. What has been studied is the beneficial effect of rhythmic movement and the resulting improvement in patients with TBI.

John is the 19-year-old competitive dancer I mentioned previously who had been in a horrific car accident. He was in a coma and suffered severe head trauma. His speech and thinking were slowed, he had a left-sided weakness, and his doctors and therapists doubted he would ever walk normally, much less dance. However, after three months, he was back doing West Coast Swing. He persevered, and his athletic abilities improved his speech and thinking. Three years later, he was better than ever. He attributes his remarkable improvement to his work and love of dance. When asked what dance means to him, he smiles, *"Dance is my passion, my motivation, my future."*

A small, landmark study is looking at movement and improvement with TBI. Dr. Corene Hurt studied eight patients, post-injury.

She and her group measured their ability to walk symmetrically and to the rhythm of the music. They also measured their speed of walking. After training to music daily for five weeks, five of the patients improved significantly.[49]

Researchers are now looking at using dance to help improve TBI since, through studies of other neurologic conditions we know it can improve physical and cognitive function. The key is to find a therapy that works and helps patients to stay with it.

Getting patients to go to physical therapy and rehab regularly is often challenging. Having an activity they enjoy is a great motivator to help them heal their brains. Many studies show that the enjoyment factor of exercise influences long-term participation.[50]

Another treatment that appears to help is Hyperbaric Oxygen therapy. Patients sit or lay in a chamber that provides 100% oxygen for 90 minutes. Treatments take 2 hours total in the hyperbaric chamber, a tube-like structure. They are administered on consecutive days, and most patients require 20 treatments. Insurance covers some conditions. Out-of-pocket cost is $250-300 a session.[51]

I spoke to a patient who had TBI that occurred while serving in the military in Afghanistan. He suffered from PTSD, tinnitus (ringing in the ears), insomnia, and migraines. After 40 sessions, he noted improved sleep, brain function, and a reduction in migraine headaches. His tinnitus is not gone completely but has been reduced by 50 percent. This is a dramatic improvement for him.

THE WRAP UP FOR BRAIN 101

If you become a partner in your body's health, you will see how you can protect your brain and keep it healthy!

• • •

Become a good partner for yourself.

• • •

The brain NEEDS fat. For starters, I told you the brain is 60% fat. If you cut all the fat out of your diet, you may note you get a little loopy. Choose GOOD, healthy fats such as Omega 3 fatty acids and plant-based fats such as that from avocados.

Show your brain some TLC. As I discussed, the brain needs healthy foods, relaxation with meditation, and proper minerals and vitamins. There is compelling evidence that this may help prevent Alzheimer's or perhaps slow the progression.

Read, do puzzles, and take up tango or martial arts.

Find dance classes in your area and just start.

Your brain needs stimulation. Feed it with wonderful information and interactions. If you don't use it, you will lose it.

Don't smoke. Your brain needs a good blood supply. You can have a stroke if you deprive it of that by smoking or having blood pressure that is out of control or cholesterol plugging up the arteries.

For those with Parkinson's or Alzheimer's, check into TMS centers and find out what new possibilities are available such as fecal transplant.

Check out Rock Steady Boxing and Shout Out! If you have Parkinson's disease.

And Check out HBOT for TBI if you are suffering as a result.

Partner with your doctor

Talk to your doctor to ensure optimal minerals and vitamin levels.

Vitamin D levels between 40ng/ml and 80 ng/ml are optimal. Most people can safely take 1000 IU of vitamin D daily. Have your zinc and magnesium levels checked.

Some diseases can mimic Alzheimer's disease. They include hypothyroidism and Lyme disease. Please make sure you are checked for these if you are having any issues. All you need are simple blood tests for this.

• • •

If you are not an exerciser,

get a stress test before you start to push yourself.

• • •

To take care of your brain, you MUST take care of your heart. Your brain needs oxygen delivered by the heart and the blood vessels. Keep your brain in good shape by keeping your heart in good condition!

CHAPTER 2

THE HEART

The heart is one of organs we often take for granted. As long as it's running okay, we don't pay much attention. Ah, but it is hard to ignore when it suddenly stops working well.

I have a patient, Fred, who called me one morning. He was a marathon runner and incredibly fit. He ate well and came for preventive visits, so I knew something was really off when he told me he was out of breath just walking up a few stairs. I told him to go to the emergency room, but he didn't want to because he had no pain. So, I had him come in to see me immediately and met him in the waiting room with a wheelchair. The room was empty and quiet, except for a soft *whoosh* sound. *Whoosh. Whoosh. Whoosh.* I could hear his heart without a stethoscope and knew then what had probably happened to him. I placed my stethoscope on Fred's chest, listened, and told him he was going right over to the cardiac unit.

I suspected he ruptured the papillary muscle connecting one of his heart valves to a portion of the heart called the trabeculae carneae that lines the ventricle of the heart. Fred's valve was flailing in his heart, and that was the noise I heard. He stood up from the wheelchair. "Just where do you think you're going?" I asked. He thought he would leave my office and walk across the street to the hospital. NO WAY. I convinced him of the gravity of his condition, and after some cajoling, he allowed himself to be rushed to the emergency room via ambulance. The thought of his trying to walk there almost gave *me* a heart attack! He could have collapsed along the way due to heart failure. My suspicions were correct; Fred had ruptured his heart valve. It took him a while, but now he is back to running marathons.

Fred's case was an example of an event that could *not* be ignored. But, often, people don't notice subtle changes in exercise tolerance or disregard twinges of pain they think are muscular and just an annoyance. We tend to discount our own symptoms because we can't believe anything bad could happen to us, but it can and does. The heart deserves our respect and our attention. We must take care of it, or it will no longer take care of us.

– HEART 101–

The heart is incredible. I was awed when I first saw a live heart beating in a patient's chest. It is miraculous and beautiful. The heart is the pump made of muscle that powers our body. It weighs about 11 ounces and beats approximately 100,000 times a day. It has a complex electrical system that keeps our heart and body moving to a steady beat. The pace of the beat, as we already learned, is dictated by the brain. The heart's purpose is to remove deoxygenated blood from the body, pump it to the lungs for oxygen, receive it back from the lungs, and then send the oxygenated blood back into the body after feeding itself by supplying blood to the coronary arteries.

There are two upper chambers known as the atria and two lower chambers known as the ventricles. Blood from the body is returned through the venous system to the heart, where it arrives at the right atrium. From there, it goes through the tricuspid valve to the right ventricle, which pumps the blood to the lungs. The blood lets go of carbon dioxide from the used blood that was returned and receives oxygen. It is pumped back to the left atrium, then pumped into the left ventricle through the mitral valve and out into the body through the aortic valve.

Keeping an eye on the health of your heart is essential throughout your lifetime. And when it comes to measuring the heart's health, the three biggies are blood pressure, pulse, and respiratory rate. Along with body temperature, these measurements are known as your vital signs, and for a good reason—they are the indicators of your body's most critical functions.

First, let's talk about blood pressure. We're all familiar with the term, and nearly everyone has had their doctor take their blood pressure, but what exactly does it mean?

When we use a blood pressure monitor, we are given a reading of two numbers. The top number is the systolic blood pressure. This indicates the pressure exerted against the arterial walls to push the blood forward from the heart to send oxygenated blood to the body. The bottom number is diastolic pressure, which indicates the pressure against the arterial walls as your heart rests and the ventricles or bottom chambers of the heart fill. The measurement is in millimeters of mercury.

Our blood pressure naturally rises with age, obesity, fatty diets, and poor exercise habits, which are major cardiac risk factors. Normal blood pressure is less than 120/80 mm Hg. But as our blood vessels stiffen with age or become thicker from the build-up of cholesterol or inflammation, they get tougher and narrower, and more force is needed to push blood through them. Your blood pressure is classified as elevated when your systolic blood pressure is between 120 to 129, and your diastolic pressure remains below 80 mm Hg.

Persistently elevated blood pressure above a certain point is called hypertension, and it's a serious problem. Hypertension puts a lot of stress on your body, particularly the heart, and is one of the leading causes of life-threatening heart failure and stroke. Hypertension stage 1 is when blood pressure consistently ranges from 130 to 139 systolic and 80 to 89 diastolic. Hypertension stage 2 is when blood pressure is consistently in the 140/90 range or higher. At this point, your doctor may advise treatment.[1]

A hypertensive crisis occurs when a sudden increase in blood pressure is greater than 180/120 mm Hg. This usually warrants a trip to the emergency room or at least a call to your doctor. If it is accompanied by chest pain, shortness of breath, vision, or speech changes, don't wait. Call 911.

The World Health Organization considers hypertension the most important preventable risk factor for death in the world. So, everyone must monitor their blood pressure and make preventive lifestyle choices to avoid developing hypertension. Blood pressure needs to be regularly monitored by your doctor, but pharmacies and community health centers often have free devices to measure blood pressure.

Next is your pulse, or heart rate, the rate at which your heart pumps. The beat that occurs when you aren't active is your resting heart rate or RHR. A normal RHR is between 60 and 100, although athletes with conditioned hearts may have an RHR lower than 60. RHR can vary a fair bit depending on surrounding conditions. For example, heat can increase your pulse by about 10 beats a minute. Body position can change it, too, especially when you go from lying to standing. Emotions can raise your pulse, and innumerable medications also affect heart rate. Those that block adrenaline, such as beta-blockers, slow the heart. Amphetamines and excessive thyroid medication will speed it up.

There are some instances when the heart's electrical system is blocked, and the pulse can drop very low. Bradycardia is the term for RHR that falls under 50-60 beats per minute. A rate this low can cause fainting or even death. If this ever happens to you, where you notice you are feeling dizzy and your pulse is low, or you have passed out, it is time to see a doctor immediately.

Conversely, if your rate is excessively fast or irregular, a condition called tachycardia, and you feel dizzy or faint, it is again time to seek help. You could have atrial fibrillation, flutter, supraventricular tachycardia, or ventricular tachycardia. These can all cause serious problems. Your pulse can easily be measured at home by placing your index and middle finger on your neck near the windpipe. When you find the pulse, count the number of beats you feel in fifteen seconds, and then multiply by four. As an interesting aside, you might wonder why no one recommends you use your thumb to check a pulse; the thumb is the only finger with its own separate blood supply. For that reason, it has its own pulse. It would make things very confusing to use it as a pulse checker.

Finally, let's discuss how oxygen gets to the heart. We describe this as your respiratory rate, how quickly you breathe. A normal respiratory rate for an adult is between 12 and 16 breaths a minute, but many conditions can alter that rate, such as asthma, heart failure, and panic.

The whole point of breathing is to deliver oxygen to the lungs, which bind with red blood cells via hemoglobin, and then travel through the heart and around the body to where it's needed. The measure of how much oxygen is in the body is called oxygen saturation. This value is the fraction of the oxygen-saturated hemoglobin relative to the total amount of hemoglobin in the blood. A healthy body is a well-oxygenated body, and the normal level is 95 to 100 percent.

Oxygen saturation will decrease if getting air into the lungs is impaired through conditions like asthma, COPD, or pneumonia. Or in trauma, where there is blood loss, the binding of oxygen to hemoglobin may be normal, but there may not be enough blood, so there is not enough oxygen. And poisons such as cyanide and carbon monoxide bind to hemoglobin and prevent oxygen from attaching.

One of the most unmistakable signs of low oxygen saturation, known as hypoxemia, is hyperventilation, or an excessive respiratory rate, as the body tries to compensate for low oxygen saturation. You must see your doctor to find the underlying cause if you regularly find yourself hyperventilating. However, mild hypoxemia may simply cause discomfort or shortness of breath that may be ignored yet can be a warning sign of a serious or developing cardiac or respiratory condition.

These days it is easy to monitor your oxygen saturation with inexpensive monitors found at most pharmacies. There are also free phone apps.

The heart doesn't act alone. It works in concert with your brain and gut to keep your body moving and grooving to a healthy beat.

We Know How the Heart Connects With the Brain, What About the Gut?

The gut-heart connection is based in the microbiome. The microbiome, as we've already discussed, is genetic material, including bacteria, fungi, protozoa, and viruses. It consists of 39 trillion microbial cells, the majority of which are in our gut and stool. The microbiome can weigh between three and five pounds and is often considered another organ. It regulates the manufacture of certain vitamins and hormones and even our immune system and weight. So, you might ask, where does the heart come into this?

Research in 2020 found that when the balance of gut bacteria is off, it can cause all kinds of problems. These include depression, autoimmune disease, obesity, *and* damage to the blood vessels and heart. This imbalance has been associated with a higher risk of heart failure, hardening of the arteries, and heart attack.[2]

The Vagus Nerve as the Wanderer

I talked about the vagus nerve and the heart in BRAIN 101. As you recall, the vagus nerve can slow the heart rate. I confess that I have an occasional heart rhythm abnormality called supraventricular tachycardia or SVT. If I am nervous or my heart rate gets too high, I will develop an uncomfortably rapid regular rhythm. My heart will race so fast that I get dizzy, and I have to sit down and/or lie down. Over the years, I've learned how to utilize the vagus nerve to break the SVT. If I put my face in ice water or hold my breath and bear down or cough, I can get it to stop. These are called vagal maneuvers which stimulate the nerve to do its thing and slow the heart down.

The bottom line is that the heart is the primary feeder of your organs. If it is not working correctly, nothing else will either. We need oxygen to survive, and that is what the heart is doing, pumping oxygen.

To feel good, the heart needs to be in healthy working order. If it's not, you could be in big trouble.

A Healthy Heart Leads to a Healthy Body

Do you know the signs of a heart attack? If not, you better learn because time is muscle. The quicker you improve blood supply the less likely you are to have it destroyed, and its destruction can kill you.

Heart attacks occur when blood is unable to get to the heart muscle and you need immediate medical care. You and your heart can be saved, but getting to the hospital as fast as possible is essential. Most hospitals that care for cardiac patients will have you assessed and treated within thirty minutes—opening the blockage or bypassing the blocked vessels to return blood flow to your heart. The sooner you are treated, the more likely you are to come out on the other side without damage. Knowing how to spot a heart attack can save a life.

The number-one killer of men and women is heart disease. According to the Centers for Disease Control, there are around 690,000 deaths yearly in the United States alone due to heart disease. That is the equivalent of one out of every four deaths! Fortunately, many heart problems are preventable. By knowing how to care for your heart and keep it healthy, you can avoid becoming a statistic.[3]

How To Save a Life (Your Own)

Joan was a 68-year-old woman with diabetes and high blood pressure. One evening she experienced intense nausea, heartburn, neck pressure, and a sense of impending doom. She drove to the emergency room, where she was asked to take a seat. Joan waited quietly for three hours, during which time her condition deteriorated. When doctors finally got to her, she was clammy and weak and her blood pressure had dropped precipitously. Joan suffered a heart attack right there in the waiting room. And although she eventually recovered, Joan's heart sustained permanent damage that might have been avoided if she had recognized the symptoms and responded appropriately—by calling an ambulance and demanding medical assistance.

Many public service announcements and educational materials are circulated to help Americans understand how to recognize and prevent heart disease. Unfortunately, many people still don't get it. In 2014, a large study found only 42.7% of the respondents could identify the five major warning signs of a heart attack. This is particularly pertinent to women and those caring for women, since their signs of heart attack can be more subtle and can sneak up on them.[4]

Chest Pain

This can be severe chest pain or pressure, like an elephant sitting on your chest. In women, however, it can be as mild as discomfort or indigestion. A couple of my female patients felt a vague chest pain or ache that was hard to describe. One felt it on the left and the other in the middle. Neither found relief with antacids or acid blocker medications. It made them anxious, but it was not a panic attack. Panic attacks go away within minutes, and this discomfort did not. That ought to be a clue it is something more ominous than heartburn.

Pain in the Arms and Shoulder

This does not always occur. When it does, many people dismiss it, thinking they may have slept wrong or lifted something heavy. The pain is usually more of an ache than a soreness. It is often described as an overwhelming feeling of weakness, and in many it will occur while exercising.

Pain in the Jaw, Neck, or Back

Several of my female patients complained only of jaw pain while having a heart attack. Both went to the dentist thinking it was a toothache. What they failed to mention to the dentists were the symptoms they did not want to acknowledge: accompanying fatigue and total body weakness that were also present with the pain. This should have been a tip-off that it was more than just a toothache.

Shortness of Breath

When the onset is unexplained, it arouses concern. Continued shortness of breath accompanied by fatigue or discomfort ought to set off alarm bells that the heart is in jeopardy. In addition, patients may experience overwhelming fatigue, nausea, sweating, anxiety or uneasiness, and a sense of impending doom.

Feeling Dizzy or Lightheaded

I had a patient who experienced severe nausea, vomiting, and dizziness along with the above symptoms. She was sure she had food poisoning. Rather than getting better after her violent spells, she continued to weaken until she finally collapsed and was sent to the ER. Food poisoning doesn't continue like that; if you experience prolonged GI symptoms, see a doctor.

• • •

Listen to your body and trust your gut.

• • •

DON'T WAIT. If you have any of the above symptoms, *listen to your body and trust your gut.* Intuition is a powerful thing. If you think something serious is going on, you are probably correct. Call 911 immediately. Time is of the essence. While waiting for the ambulance chew a 325 mg aspirin (unless you are allergic to it). That will help thin the blood and potentially improve the blocked artery causing the pain.

Evaluate Your Risk

There are a variety of risk factors that can increase the chances of having a heart attack. Some are genetic, and others are very preventable. The classic genetic factors that put you at risk for hardening of the arteries and heart attack include:

- a family history of heart disease in a first-degree relative (mother, father, sister, or brother);

- increasing age;

- men are at higher risk at first; women catch up after menopause;

- high cholesterol or increased lipids or fats in the blood (these tend to be hereditary);

- high blood pressure (which can be genetic as well).

Take your cardiac risk factors seriously! One of the things we hear about all the time is the importance of managing our risk factors for heart disease. Unfortunately, the dangers of *not* doing that are not sinking in. Sure, we *may* know what to do in an acute event like a heart attack. That is a scary, dramatic event. However, the idea of heart disease becoming chronic doesn't occur to most.

Many moons ago, when I started in practice, I thought hospice care was reserved for cancer patients. It wasn't until I saw a patient enter hospice care for debilitating heart disease that I realized it could be a terminal, chronic disease and equally as deadly as cancer.

Heart failure, irreversible coronary disease, and severe arrhythmias can be disabling. If you can't walk across a room or be active in any way, you have a problem. Some people give up. They may be resigned to having coronary or heart disease. They may not want or be offered procedures to help. Most do not realize that

• • •

it is possible to reverse disease on your own.

• • •

Dr. Dean Ornish conducted several programs to reverse coronary disease by following a particular lifestyle plan. As early as 1977, he showed improved blood flow to the heart in only one month. A randomized control trial in 1983 confirmed that heart function improved in one month *and,* he showed that severe coronary artery blockages could reverse in just a year. His five-year findings published in 1998 showed an average improvement in the heart of more than 300% and a decrease in cardiac events by 2.5 times.[5]

The diet in the Ornish program focuses on reducing the intake of high-fat meats and full-fat dairy. The consumption of complex carbohydrates such as fruits, veggies, whole grains, legumes, non-fat dairy, soy products, and egg whites is encouraged. Moderate amounts of fish, avocados, nuts, seeds, and skinless chicken are also part of the diet. The prevention diet (keeping heart disease from forming) is less strict than the diet to reverse coronary disease. To reverse disease, the Ornish plan reduces the consumption of fat calories to just 10 percent with less than 10 milligrams of cholesterol a day. Is this safe? Actually, studies have found that it is.

The Ornish plan isn't just about what you eat. As in the Blue Zones (which you will hear about later), it is also about lifestyle.

Exercise is essential and needs to be part of daily life. Ornish recommends at least twenty minutes a day of aerobic activity.

Stress management is important and can include stretching, breathing exercises, imagery, and meditation.

Social support is also necessary. Spending time with family, friends, and community promotes healthy hearts.[6]

Knowing that you have control over what happens to your arteries by managing the all-important cardiac risk factors, here is what you need to know.

Factors You Can Change:

- Elevated Cholesterol
- Hypertension
- Obesity
- A sedentary lifestyle
- Tobacco use
- Diabetes
- Stress

- Depression
- Loneliness
- History of autoimmune disease
- TMAO (Trimethylamine N-oxide
  —*more on this shortly*)

I wanted to include a statistic that shows the percentage of risk for developing heart disease concerning each of the above factors. However, it is impossible due to the fact that each condition has varying severity levels. So, the risks will be individual. In addition, risks often may be clustered in combinations. For instance, people who are overweight or obese often have type 2 diabetes and high cholesterol. I have referenced the risk factors individually so that you can explore them if you like.[7-17]

What Can You Do?

Obviously, you cannot prevent aging or change your genetics. But there are things you can control. First: become informed. Have your blood pressure checked annually, along with your cholesterol and fasting blood sugar. Check your weight, as many people who are overweight or obese do not recognize (or admit) they have an issue. Extra poundage adds additional risk for diabetes, heart disease, stroke, certain cancers, and various other problems. If you would like an actual number that shows your risk, there is an app for that! It is free. Go to ASCVD Risk Estimator. You will be asked your age, gender, race, systolic blood pressure, and high blood pressure treatment and if you are a smoker and/or a diabetic. It will also ask for your total cholesterol and HDL cholesterol. These values are obtained from a simple blood test by your doctor called a lipid panel.

Check Your Cholesterol

When measuring cholesterol, I usually recommend a one-time blood test that measures the actual cholesterol particles. Most physicians do not do this test routinely, but I find it very helpful. It is called the NMR lipoprofile study which shows the actual value of your LDL or "bad cholesterol." The usual lipid profile *calculates* the bad or LDL cholesterol using an equation: LDL cholesterol = Total Cholesterol – HDL (the good cholesterol) – Triglycerides/5. It gives a numerical value of your cholesterol level, but it will not show you the whole picture, as other particles may help predict the risk of heart disease.[18]

The type of cholesterol you have matters. There are different types of LDL. There are the large particles, big and fluffy and not as toxic as the small particle type, which is dense and can eat away at arteries and cause plaque. There are two types of HDL cholesterol: type 2, which is large and protective, and type 3, which is not as protective. You could have high LDL levels, but if they're big and fluffy they probably won't cause you any problems, but if they're small and dense, you've got an issue.

In my opinion, the NMR test is far more helpful to see if your cholesterol levels need to be treated with medication. I am more likely to recommend a cholesterol-lowering drug to a patient with small dense LDL particles and low HDL 2 levels. In addition, because everything is measured in this test, I can see what a patient's triglyceride levels look like when they are non-fasting. This can be very helpful because high triglycerides (fasting or not) can increase the risk of an inflamed pancreas. If the test is done fasting, it can show an increased risk for insulin resistance or metabolic syndrome. Metabolic syndrome is defined by a group of problems, including high blood pressure, increased blood sugar, and fat around the middle leading to an increased risk for heart disease. It's not enough to just know your numbers; you need to understand what they mean.

Check Your Blood Pressure

If you have high blood pressure in the doctor's office, check your blood pressure at home. I have many patients who have high blood pressure only in my office, but it is because either I make them nervous or just being in a doctor's office makes them anxious, causing a momentary blood pressure rise. They do not need to be on medication. If there is any question regarding what time of day their blood pressure is elevated, I use a 24–hour blood pressure monitor that the patient wears at home. It records blood pressure throughout the day. This has been enormously helpful for my patients. Ask your doctor about one of these devices if you think you may have variable blood pressure related to stressful situations.

A nurse I care for, Cheryl, is a great example of unusual blood pressure elevations due to stress. She became alarmed when someone at work checked her blood pressure and found it was sky-high. She wondered if she needed medication. The 24–hour monitor showed that her blood pressure was only high at work when she was assigned to a particular doctor. She made some changes at work and is no longer working with that person. Now no more high blood pressure—problem solved! Sometimes you have to look beyond the obvious. Widen the scope, because there are a lot of factors that play into heart disease.

One of the most common pieces of advice for people with high blood pressure or other risk factors for heart disease, such as high cholesterol, obesity, and sedentary behavior, is to exercise. Yet, few patients actually follow this advice. The problem is that it is tough to get people to do it. A patient of mine found a fun way to deal with his cardiac risk factors. Phil is a 60-year-old Filipino man diagnosed with high blood pressure and was on medication. Five years ago, he started partner dancing. His doctor noted that his blood pressure was lower each year than before until his blood pressure medication was finally wholly discontinued. His weight and blood pressure have decreased, and he is feeling fantastic.

Since exercise is vital for high blood pressure control, several studies have been conducted to see if something is fun and entertaining enough to get people moving and keep them moving. A 2013 study published by the Centers for Disease Control found nearly 80% of Americans do not get their recommended exercise. Researchers surveyed 450,000 adults in the United States over the age of 18. About 23% of all the men and 18% of the women met the recommended exercise requirements. People between 18 and 24 were most likely to exercise, and those over 65 were least likely to exercise.[19]

Scientists have looked at what motivates us to move. Further studies have found those who have fun exercising are more likely to engage in it.[3,20] The key is to find a way for it to be enjoyable. One of those ways is to engage in ballroom dance. Multiple studies looking at a variety of dances including Cha-Cha, Rumba, Salsa, and Tango have been found to lower blood pressure and heart rates and improve heart function when done regularly. Exercise can do this as well, but ballroom dancers are far more likely to dance regularly because it is social and fun.

Quit Smoking

Tobacco use is a major risk factor for heart disease and stroke and needs to be stopped, and preferably never started. The moment you stop, your risk diminishes.

A cohort study published in 2022 examined smoking and smoking cessation associated with mortality risks.[21] The study included 500,000 adults in the US National Health Interview Survey. They noted smoking status as "current," "former," or "never smoked." They also noted when the people in the study quit and for how many years they had not smoked after quitting. Smokers more than doubled their risk of dying prematurely, while quitting was associated with an impressively reduced mortality.

One of the most remarkable things as a true testament to how well the body can heal itself, is that quitting before age 45 was associated with reductions of approximately 90% of excess mortality risk. When quitting between the ages of 45 and 64, roughly 66% of the excess risk was reduced. These statistics cannot be ignored. The sooner people stop, the better the results. The younger they are when they quit, the greater the health benefits. Those who quit before age 35 avoided almost *all* excess mortality due to smoking.

The bottom line is,

if you smoke, quit! The sooner, the better!

Yes, it is very hard to quit smoking, but millions have done it. Today there are many things available to help. There are nicotine patches, gums and inhalers, and even medications for extreme cases. There are smoking cessation groups. Hypnosis and acupuncture help as well. If you are still smoking, make it a priority to free yourself and save your body from this horribly dangerous (and expensive) habit.

Get Moving

Sitting all day can be just as bad as smoking. In fact, sitting has been referred to as the "new smoking."[22] It can be just as deleterious to your heart and overall health! The moment you start moving regularly, your health improves. A small pedal bike placed under a desk has been found to help with weight loss and make exercise possible even while sitting.

Adopt a Healthy Lifestyle

Diabetes can destroy your body. The primary cause of type 2 diabetes is obesity. Exercise, a healthy diet, and general movement throughout the day can all help improve blood sugar and prevent diabetes. Later, I will present suggestions for eating and exercise that will make you feel healthier and full of energy. These same suggestions will help with loneliness, stress, and depression, all of which can contribute to the development of heart disease. As far as autoimmune disease goes, an anti-inflammatory diet known as the Mediterranean diet can help, which we will discuss in Chapter 9.

TMAO

What about TMAO (mentioned in our risk-factor list)? TMAO stands for trimethylamine N-oxide, and you don't want too much of it in your body. Researchers from the Cleveland Clinic identified it in 2016 as a potent risk factor for heart disease and stroke. Through multiple studies, they have found when we eat foods high in L-carnitine and choline, the organisms in our gut metabolize them into trimethylamine N-oxide (TMAO). This chemical causes inflammation and narrowing of blood vessels that can reduce blood flow, which can lead to heart attack and stroke. Red meat is particularly high in L-carnitine, and farm-raised fish and egg yolks are high in choline. As noted above, this discovery is relatively recent, and recommendations in the future will be forthcoming. In the meantime, I recommend my patients have a fasting TMAO level test. This is available through the Cleveland Heart Lab. If levels are over 6.2 mM (this unit is a laboratory measure of TMAO concentration in the blood and stands for micromoles), I recommend they eliminate or decrease their consumption of red meat. In general, I urge my patients to eat only wild-caught fish. As far as egg yolks go, those with high TMAO levels probably need to limit their consumption or switch to egg whites. If elevated TMAO is a problem, food such as grape seed extract, extra virgin olive oil, and (believe it or not!) Guinness Stout can lower levels.[23]

What Is the Deal?

There is constant chatter regarding the risk factors for heart attack and heart disease. I am not sure why the message is not being received. One reason is that, despite knowing the signs, we tend to think a heart attack will not happen to us. Women, in particular, ignore the symptoms. We keep on going, doing what we do, which is usually taking care of everyone else first before taking care of ourselves.

• • •

But remember, you cannot take care of anyone if you

are not here.

• • •

Joan, the patient who sat in the ER waiting room and had a heart attack while awaiting care, did not heed that advice. After her hospitalization, her diabetes worsened, she was too busy to exercise, and she was too busy to shop for healthy foods. Three years after her heart attack, she died of a stroke. That is why understanding your risks, doing something to decrease them, and finding a lifestyle that maximizes your health is so important. Please take this advice to heart; I wish Joan had.

What Is the Deal?

A stroke can be devastating. It can occur when an artery in the brain gets blocked. This is called an ischemic stroke. It can also happen if a blood vessel in the brain ruptures and bleeds, a hemorrhagic stroke. Regardless of the cause, it is crucial to recognize the signs and get to the hospital as fast as you can. There is an acronym to help remember what to look for if someone is having a stroke: "**FAST**."[24]

- **F**ace: Look at their face and see if it is symmetrical. Is their smile drooping or their tongue going off to the side when they stick it out?

- **A**rms: Can they raise both arms, or is one dropped down?

- **S**peech: Have them repeat a phrase. Is it slurred or garbled?

- **T**ime: If the answer is yes to any of these, call 911

Time is of the essence. There are medications and procedures that can be brain-saving but need to be done very early in the evolution of a stroke. The best way to avoid a stroke is to prevent it from happening! The same risk factors we discussed for heart disease apply to strokes.

By keeping your blood pressure, cholesterol, and TMAO levels in check, not smoking, managing your stressors, avoiding diabetes, and finding a healthy weight, you can help prevent a stroke.

What Can You Do If You Have Had A Stroke?

If you have had a stroke, fear not. Many people can recover from a stroke. Speech therapy, physical therapy, and occupational therapy all help. Alternative treatments are also becoming more mainstream.

A specialized optometrist known as a neuro-optometrist can help patients regain visual function, memory, and balance with the help of special eye exercises. The results are amazing, and the treatment is non-invasive.

Recently stroke patients have been treated with hyperbaric oxygen therapy. This is where the patient sits or lies down in a tank with windows and 100% oxygen is pumped in. Patients are treated for 40 to 60 daily sessions for 90 minutes each. A study in 2020 found significant improvement in all cognitive abilities, even in late chronic stages of stroke. This result is impressive. The price tag can be high, but some insurances may pay for the treatment.[25]

So, even if all your preventive measures fail and you wind up having a stroke, there is hope for recovery.

THE WRAP-UP FOR HEART 101

In my experience as a physician and as an observer of those around me, It seems that as we get older, we often think that we don't have to keep up our fitness regimens.

We know from recent studies that increasing physical activity in those over 60 decreases the risk of heart disease by 11%. When people stop working out, their risk goes up 27%. It is never too late to start exercising; you certainly don't want to stop. I have seen it happen too often that patients come to me and let themselves go. They stop exercising and eating healthily. They are always shocked when I put them on the treadmill and check for potential heart problems, and I find them.[26]

Ironically, our ancestors had no choice but to be active and careful with what they ate, but they did not have modern medicine. We have the opposite problem. With modern medicine, amenities, and tempting foods, we do not have to work to farm and provide for ourselves. The truth is that being healthy takes work. In this day and age with modern conveniences, we must be mindful of everything we need to do to maintain it. So, here is my advice: Become a good partner to yourself and protect your heart!

Eat a healthy diet and stick to it. The Mediterranean diet is yummy, and research has confirmed over and over again that it is good for your heart.

Exercise. It is important to work out or *just move* for life. Walking is great exercise, and so is dance. Find something that is fun and heart healthy.

Never smoke, or quit if you do. Smoking is deadly—and that includes secondhand smoke. Over time, a smoking habit damages almost every part of your body. However, once you stop, the body heals.

Learn how to de-stress and deal with loneliness. Loneliness and social isolation are killers. Lonely people tend to neglect healthy habits and become depressed. (More information in chapter 6)

Stress can be powerful when it comes to the heart. Broken heart syndrome is a phenomenon that occurs after a severe stressor or trauma. Patients experience a massive outpouring of stress hormones that include adrenaline. It acts as a stun gun to the heart and looks like a heart attack. However, despite a slight elevation in cardiac enzymes, there is no evidence of a heart attack. If given supportive care, patients recover. The same thing can happen with positive stress, known as "happy heart" syndrome. It can be seen when people win a giant lottery jackpot or walk into their own surprise party.

Monitor your blood pressure and keep it in check. You cannot feel high blood pressure, so it is essential to check it regularly. My father had undiagnosed hypertension for years. He was so stubborn and refused to have it checked. It killed him. He died of kidney failure. Remember his story as a cautionary tale: high blood pressure is a silent killer.

Achieve a healthy weight to avoid Type 2 diabetes. Diabetes causes serious heart problems in addition to other issues. Maintaining a healthy weight will help to prevent it in the first place.

Put on your dancing shoes! Moving your body is essential to your heart's health.

Don't be hard on yourself if you can't do it all at once. Making these new, healthier habits stick may take a few attempts. Especially when it comes to giving up smoking. That is OK. The more times you try, the more likely you are to succeed. Don't give up.

Know the signs of a heart attack and stroke. The sooner you get help, the sooner you save your heart. Time is muscle and brainpower.

Partner with your doctor. Have he, or she follow your:

- Blood pressure

- Cholesterol

- Fasting TMAO levels. This may not be easy because many doctors don't know about it. However, they can easily get the order form and instructions from the Cleveland Clinic Heart Lab. It can be done at your local lab and costs $6.00.

- Check your fitness levels with a stress test.

- Find out your coronary calcium score with a CT angiogram.

- Discuss anxiety levels, which doctors recommend exploring in those under 65.

The heart feeds the entire body, including the gut, and the gut nourishes the heart. Without the proper nutrients or if there is an imbalance, the heart can stop. This interconnection and interdependence are essential for a healthy body and life. When it comes to keeping things going,

• • •

YOU are in the driver's seat.
I know you have the "GUTS" for that!

• • •

CHAPTER THREE

THE GUT

Chances are that most people reading this book have experienced gut issues, be it vomiting from food poisoning, heartburn after a spicy meal, or diarrhea from a foreign visit (such as Montezuma's Revenge). Gut issues are uncomfortable, to say the least. They're embarrassing, too! And that's probably why we didn't talk about them until recently. But we need to talk about the gut.

The gut or gastrointestinal system (GI) is enormous, encompassing the liver, pancreas, small and large intestines, esophagus, and stomach: a lot of organs to keep in check! Each year there are roughly 105 million ambulatory care visits and 14 million hospital admissions, and 236,000 deaths related to the GI tract. As our population ages, these numbers will only increase.

As it stands, numerous issues were elucidated in a large study by the National Institute of Health. A survey conducted of over 60,000 people across the US revealed that almost two-thirds of the Americans surveyed were burdened by gut problems. And the effects of these issues can diminish the quality and even reduce the quantity of your life. But the health of your gut isn't just a matter of comfort and avoiding problems; a healthy gut can improve your life, overall health, and even the sharpness of your thinking! The more we learn, I would go so far as to say a healthy gut is *essential* for a healthy life.[1]

The gut is considered the second brain, because it communicates through its own nervous system and, through the vagus nerve, transmits emotion and information to the brain and the rest of the body, including the heart. Although the brain is the *ultimate* command center of the body, the gut has the power to establish the overall well-being of your body and mind.[2]

It can maintain the health of your organs by protecting your immunity and preventing depression and disease. As we continue to learn more about the gut and the microbiome, I have realized that, as Hippocrates, the father of western medicine, stated over 2400 years ago, "All disease begins in the gut." That is why it is essential to respect the literal boundaries of the gut and protect them by keeping it as healthy as possible. So much is possible with the gut:

Mood Regulation (and Dysregulation): It can be the "seat" of anxiety. If a person has stomach or intestinal distress, the gut can send messages to the brain and cause emotional distress. If there is an imbalance, serotonin levels can drop and depression can occur. Researchers are discovering certain bacteria associated with different mood disorders. For example, in those with bipolar disorder and major depressive disorder, Actinobacteria Enterobacteriaceae was increased, and Faecalibacterium was decreased. This sets up a promising treatment avenue for those suffering from these disorders.[3]

Hormone Balance: Having trouble with your hormones? An imbalance in gut microbiota may be the problem. Current research shows that estrogen regulation occurs in the gut. Poor gut health can lead to polycystic ovarian syndrome, endometriosis, and even breast cancer. Even more fascinating is that cancer has its own microbiome. It promotes tumor growth, the ability to evade the body's immune system and its response to treatment.[4]

Improve Your Immune System: Since eighty percent of the immune cells in the body are located in the gut, it has a massive impact on immune function. Autoimmune disease is more likely to occur when the gut is not healthy and "leaks," as in leaky gut syndrome. I will discuss this further later in this chapter. The diseases we discussed in the brain chapter are also more likely in the face of an unhealthy gut.

Prevent Illness: The almighty gut has the power to cause illness if it is not balanced, but it also has tremendous power to heal and prevent illness. Learn how to harness that power. You can do it! Know your gut and what keeps it happy! Because if you do, you can prevent these problems and live a very long and healthy life.[1] Basically, we get our nutrition from food broken down by the gut. Nutrients enter the bloodstream and are delivered beautifully when our digestive system is healthy. Our gut contains a variety of bacteria, fungi, protozoa, viruses, and immune cells. As part of a fine-tuned machine, they all work to establish and maintain your health.

– GUT 101 –

The Gut As The Provider

Plainly said, the gut keeps us alive. It is the primary provider of nutrition and all the building blocks we need for a healthy life. We consume food, which is delivered via the esophagus to the stomach. From there it enters the small intestine which is twenty-two feet long and passes through the large intestine or colon which is five feet long. Along the way, help is provided by various organs that aid digestion and absorption of nutrients via hormones (insulin from the pancreas), enzymes (from the liver and gallbladder), and the manufacture of certain vitamins (the microbiome).

The Gut As The Great Communicator

I bet it blew your mind (pardon the pun) when I told you at the start of this chapter that the gut is considered the second brain. There are 200-600 million neurons or brain cells in your gut, accounting for ninety percent of your body's serotonin! Serotonin regulates your mood, and low levels are associated with depression. The gut is in direct communication to the brain through the vagus nerve. The vagus nerve is the tenth cranial nerve and goes from the brainstem at the base of the brain through the neck and chest and into the abdomen. Because of its path, it has been described as the "wanderer nerve." This helps to explain why we sometimes get diarrhea when we are nervous or feel butterflies in our stomach when we are excited.[5] I think it also might explain nausea that occurs with migraines.

Happy Gut, Happy Butt

Because the gut performs so many vital functions, it is important to keep it happy. Otherwise, your health can take a treacherous turn. There are obvious things, such as limiting alcohol to protect your liver (or, as my GI doctor husband says, "Love your liver!"). Watch your carbohydrate intake and weight to protect your liver and pancreas and prevent diabetes. Avoid a high-fat diet to keep your gallbladder from becoming inflamed or forming stones and pay attention to what might be bothering your GI system. Are there certain foods that cause you distress? Does spicy food give you heartburn? Are there some things you find yourself shying away from because they give you gas? These are all things to pay attention to because what you eat matters to your gut. If a particular food is giving you grief, STOP eating it. The last thing you want is for your gut to get out of whack.

How Things Can Go Sideways

The big issue, colon cancer, can be preventable! Colon cancer is the third most diagnosed cancer in the US. Approximately 4.4% of men and 4.1% of women will be diagnosed in their lifetime. This does not need to be a death sentence. Colonoscopy screening increases the doctor's ability to find it early or when it begins as a polyp before it becomes cancer. When this happens, the five-year survival rate is 91%. Most colon cancer can be detected early, around the age of 45. However, it rarely occurs in younger people. By being aware of your symptoms and not ignoring them you can improve and possibly prolong your life.[6]

I host a medical show on NBC5 KOBI in southern Oregon every Monday. Each week, I feature a different specialist, and we answer caller questions confidentially. One Monday, I was with my husband, when a twenty-seven-year-old woman called in. She told him she had experienced rectal bleeding for months and her doctor kept treating her for hemorrhoids. My husband suggested she come to see him at his GI office, and she did. He performed a colonoscopy and found rectal cancer. Fortunately, it was early. It was treated appropriately, and she went on to have a baby a year later and now has regular screenings. This is an unusual case, but it illustrates the need to pay attention to your body and do something about it if it feels off.

· · ·

Trust your gut.

· · ·

One condition many people suffer from is irritable bowel syndrome. If you suffer from this, you will see you are not alone and there are many things you can do.

Irritable Bowel Syndrome

When life turns topsy-turvy, our digestive system sometimes follows suit. But for people with irritable bowel syndrome (IBS), there's no such thing as smooth sailing. Any day, any moment might bring abdominal discomfort, cramps, bouts of diarrhea, constipation, or all of these symptoms, along with gas and bloating. It is *not* a fun ride. The key to calming the intestinal seas is sussing out what's causing the problem. Once you round that buoy, relief is in sight.

It's hard to know how many people have IBS, since many cases go undiagnosed, but one survey found about 14% of Americans suffer from it—more than 43 million people![6] Twice as many women have it as men, and people ages 25 to 54 are most vulnerable. The triggers are variable. Certain foods such as chocolate, wheat, and vegetables can increase the symptoms. Stress also plays a significant role. Abnormal proteins have recently been found in those with IBS. Research is ongoing and the significance of these abnormal proteins is still unclear.

Not all digestive problems that seem like IBS actually are. In fact, IBS is what we call a diagnosis of exclusion, or **I Be** **S***tumped*. When all other possibilities have been ruled out, IBS is likely. To illustrate the difficulty of the IBS diagnosis, I will weave tales of three women into this chapter, all with "gut-wrenching" problems. Only one had IBS, but all three got significant relief once they found the proper treatment. Let's start with Beth.

Beth, a young woman of 26, had suffered her whole life with severe abdominal pain that came and went. She also complained of horrible gas that was particularly smelly. After talking with Beth, it seemed her symptoms worsened after she ate dairy products and fruit. I sent her to a gastroenterologist for two different breath tests.

The first, a hydrogen breath test, examined her ability to digest dairy. She was given a milk preparation to drink, then blew into special bags every twenty minutes for three hours. The bags were analyzed for the presence of hydrogen and methane. She had high levels of both, which pointed to lactose intolerance (a deficiency of lactase, the enzyme that digests milk sugars) and overgrowth in the small intestine of a type of bacteria that produces methane. We treated her with antibiotics and asked her to cut out dairy and fruit in an effort to starve the methane-producing bacteria in her gut. It worked, and she improved, but she still wasn't "right."

Next, Beth had a fructose tolerance test for her ability to digest fruit. The same procedure was repeated after she drank a fructose drink. Sure enough, she was found to also have fructose intolerance. The fructose drink stirred up her old symptoms, so we gave her another course of antibiotics to treat the bacterial overgrowth. Finally, her symptoms have resolved after a lifetime of suffering and now she knows what foods to avoid so they don't return.

Beth had food intolerances and bacterial overgrowth, but not true IBS since her symptoms resolved once the causes were eradicated.

The Foods That Ail Us: Allergies All Around

As you discovered above, many digestive problems that seem like IBS stem from food intolerance. If you have a food intolerance, in one sense you're lucky because your symptoms will most likely disappear after you cut the problem foods out of your diet. Below are some of the most common intolerances.

Lactose Intolerance

Got milk? If you do and you're lactose intolerant, you probably also have diarrhea, bloating, belly pain, and maybe even nausea. Lactose intolerance is caused by a deficiency of the enzyme lactase. Produced by the small intestine, it helps the body digest lactose, a sugar found in milk and other dairy products. (Yes, milk contains natural sugars, even before you add the chocolate syrup.) You might think you're either born lactose intolerant or not, but lactase deficiency develops over time and becomes more common with age. It can also occur after chemotherapy for cancer. People with Inflammatory bowel disease (IBD) are also at increased risk.

There are two ways to diagnose the condition. The easiest is to avoid milk products and see if your digestive problems go away. The other is to take the same breath test as Beth: First, you consume a dairy drink, then breathe into a special bag for several hours. If the hydrogen level in your breath is high, you have lactase deficiency and are lactose intolerant.

Most lactose intolerant people can tolerate a little bit of lactose and some can tolerate yogurt with active cultures (thanks to the lactase-producing "cultures," or bacteria) and/or hard cheeses. Your tolerance depends on how much or how little lactase your body produces. An enzyme supplement such as Lactaid or Similase can help you digest dairy more easily. Probiotics, including the extra-strong product VSL#3 (which requires the supervision of the doctor treating you for IBS), can also aid digestion.

Fructose Intolerance

An apple a day might help keep the doctor away, but not for someone with fructose intolerance, also known as fructose malabsorption. Some studies suggest it's a common cause of irritable bowel symptoms.[7]

Can someone really be intolerant of fruit? Unfortunately, yes, as Beth's story also illustrated. People with fructose malabsorption have trouble digesting the sugar fructose found in fruit and anything made with high fructose corn syrup. When these people eat fruit, the sugar is not fully absorbed in their small intestines, so it makes its way to the large intestine—also known as the bowel— where it doesn't belong. There it can wreak havoc, causing problems with gas, bloating, pain, and more.

Fructose intolerance can be diagnosed with another type of hydrogen breath test very similar to the lactose intolerance test. You'll be given a fructose drink and asked to blow into a bag every fifteen minutes for several hours. The test is positive if you have a lot of hydrogen in your breath. The easy treatment is to avoid fructose. You would think that would mean avoiding all fruit. Luckily, berries have minimal amounts of fructose, so are generally okay to eat. But other fruits and foods with high fructose corn syrup will cause problems.

Gluten Intolerance

If you've never noticed the proliferation of gluten-free products on grocery store shelves, you will now. It seems every other person I meet is going gluten-free. Contrary to popular belief, cutting out gluten will not help you lose weight, not any more than cutting out simple carbs in general. So, if weight loss is your objective, you might as well embrace gluten again. But some people have gluten intolerance (not to be confused with celiac disease). They may experience IBS-type symptoms after eating wheat, rye, barley, or other gluten-containing foods. For people with this intolerance, avoiding gluten will relieve their symptoms. However, if they eat some gluten occasionally, it won't hurt them, in contrast to people with celiac disease, who must not consume *any* gluten.

If you test negative for celiac disease, that doesn't mean you don't have gluten intolerance. Unfortunately, there is no definitive test for gluten intolerance. The best way to know is to avoid gluten for thirty days and see if your symptoms improve. Anna, the next patient you will read about, has celiac disease. The same foods she needs to avoid can work for those with gluten intolerance.

Celiac Disease

Anna is a 50-year-old new patient who came to see me for a physical exam. She told me she was healthy, but as we talked, I discovered Anna suffered from abdominal discomfort she hadn't thought to mention because she'd simply gotten used to having it. She had suffered intermittent bouts of diarrhea and low-level fatigue for years.

As part of her evaluation, I did a blood test to check for celiac disease. This inflammatory condition of the small intestine results from a reaction to gluten. Her test was markedly positive. In addition, all her vitamin levels were low. This wasn't a surprise since celiac disease compromises the ability of the gastrointestinal tract to absorb vitamins from food.

The treatment for her was to cut out gluten from her diet. This means avoiding not only the obvious things like most bread, pasta, cereal, crackers, and cookies but also a whole host of other food products, including most beer, baked goods, candy, French fries, gravy, imitation seafood, salad dressings, some sauces (including soy sauce), seasoned rice mixes, and some soups and seasoned snack foods, to name many but not all. Gluten is even found in some cosmetics!

Anna has been very good at avoiding these foods and is doing well. She no longer has abdominal discomfort and her energy level has skyrocketed. She is a bit upset; now that she is absorbing nutrients from food properly, she has gained ten pounds! Like Beth,

Anna didn't have IBS. Her celiac disease was the problem and a change of diet was the solution.

Anna was diagnosed with celiac disease, an autoimmune disease resulting in gluten intolerance. You might say it's the IT disease of the century. It turns out that about 1 in 140 Americans has celiac disease![8] If you do, your body attacks the cells of the small intestine when it is exposed to gluten. The result is poor absorption of nutrients leading to nutritional deficiencies.

Some people have very few symptoms. Others experience diarrhea or constipation, bloating, vitamin D deficiency, itchy skin rashes, and other autoimmune problems such as thyroiditis (inflammation of the thyroid gland). If celiac disease goes untreated, it can also cause a host of difficult or even life-threatening symptoms. These include fatigue, bone or joint pain, osteoporosis, depression, canker sores, tingling in the hands or feet, missed menstrual periods, and even infertility or frequent miscarriages. It can also result in malnutrition and anemia and increase the risk for certain cancers such as lymphoma.[9]

Celiac disease is diagnosed by a blood test and confirmed by a small bowel biopsy, which can be accomplished with an upper endoscopy by a gastroenterologist. (In this test, the doctor places a long, flexible tube with a camera at its tip down your esophagus.) The treatment is relatively simple: avoid gluten. Since the awareness of celiac disease has increased, so has the availability of gluten-free products. Celiac is an autoimmune disease. It is not considered a food allergy or food sensitivity.

True Food Allergies

There are a few major scary food allergies (shellfish, eggs, cows' milk), but the big one is peanuts. Those with this condition exposed to *anything* peanut—the nut, the oil—can die as a result. Others might have an allergic reaction and mount a response with elevated levels of the antibody IgE. There is often a reaction when these are present in certain foods, but it is not usually deadly. When I suspect these reactions in patients, I order a food allergy panel to help them see which foods are the culprits and what they need to eliminate. A patient, Gwen, just wasn't feeling good. She was tired and achy. We ordered a food allergy panel and found she was allergic to tomatoes and lettuce, her favorite health foods. Gwen did not want to believe that healthy food could cause problems. At first, she was angry with *me* and refused to change her diet. However, Gwen was desperate and, finally, she did it. When she eliminated tomatoes and lettuce, she felt she was back to her usual healthy self.

Other Causes of Cranky Bowels

When I see a patient with IBS symptoms, I ensure that they don't have gluten sensitivity, celiac disease, lactose intolerance, or fructose intolerance. I also screen for inflammatory bowel disease (IBD), colon cancer, and MTHFR mutations.

People with one or more mutations of a particular gene called MTHFR (methylenetetrahydrofolate reductase) can't process folic acid efficiently. They may feel it in their gut, since folic acid plays a role in keeping the gut happy. MTHFR *is* good when it's working correctly in the body; it helps turn folic acid into L-methylfolate, an active form of the vitamin, which the body needs to make the "feel-good" hormones serotonin, dopamine, and norepinephrine.[10] You probably think of serotonin as a brain chemical. But—surprise!—the gastrointestinal system is lined with cells that look like brain cells and they secrete serotonin, too. (See Chapter 6.)

MTHFR Mutations

This gene codes for the metabolism of folic acid. As I mentioned above, mutations in the MTHFR gene can cause the body problems with producing serotonin, which is important to the gut and the brain. If you have IBS, ask to be tested for a mutation of this gene. If you have one or more mutations, a supplement of L-methylfolate—a simple vitamin—could solve your problems.

Another cause of irritable bowels should not be missed. I am talking about Inflammatory bowel disease or IBD. Inflammatory bowel disease includes Crohn's disease and ulcerative colitis, auto-immune diseases in which the body turns on itself, involving the colon and/or the small bowel, causing severe inflammation. In addition, they create blood and mucus in the stool, pain, and often weight loss. They also increase a person's risk for colon cancer.[11] As you can imagine, the work-up for all this can get quite expensive. I often see patients with no insurance. If you'd like to investigate on your own before undergoing tests, an elimination diet is a low-cost way to rule out lactose, fructose, or gluten intolerance. If an elimination diet doesn't help, you may need a colonoscopy to rule out serious problems, including IBD and colon cancer.

IBD and Colon Cancer

IBD is an umbrella term that includes Crohn's disease and ulcerative colitis. As I explained above, people with IBD have diarrhea, cramping, mucus, and often blood in the stool. IBD also can cause unexplained weight loss.

Colon cancer can cause a change in bowel habits or there may be no symptoms. If you are typically constipated and start having frequent diarrhea, that could be a reason for concern. If you usually have diarrhea and for no apparent reason you become constipated, that's also a red flag. Some people may notice their stools are narrowing. A colonoscopy will help to identify IBD and rule out colon cancer and is usually performed before a diagnosis of IBS is given.

Bacterial Overgrowth

Bacterial overgrowth occurs when the number of bacteria in our gut increases significantly. Our stomach acid usually controls the number of bacteria, but now that many people are taking acid-blocking drugs such as Prilosec or other acid-lowering medications like Tagamet or Zantac, the bacteria numbers can grow unchecked. Also, decreased motility (movement) of the intestines due to diabetes or a disease such as IBD is another cause of overgrowth in the intestines. Poor motility allows "bad" bacteria to thrive.

Treatment addresses the underlying cause in the case of patients with motility issues or IBD. Antibiotics reduce the number of bacteria. Probiotics—supplements of "good" bacteria—help repopulate the gut with healthy bacteria, which help keep "bad" bacteria in check.

When All Your Tests Are Negative

Carol suffered from irritable bowel symptoms her whole life. But breath tests and a colonoscopy turned up nothing. During her evaluation, Carol shared her personal history with me—and it was not pretty. She grew up in a dysfunctional family and had been molested and physically and emotionally abused. She left home at fifteen. She lived on the streets for some time and had been raped and beaten. Miraculously, she was able to get her life together. She now has a thriving business and a wonderful family. However, she had disabling IBS symptoms.

I referred her to a psychologist for eye movement desensitization reprocessing (EMDR) therapy, a technique often used to treat people with post-traumatic stress disorder, and useful for anyone who's lived through traumatic stress of any sort and suffering from physical symptoms. In this therapy, a specially trained psychologist distracts your brain, either by having you follow her finger with your eyes or by making tapping or other sounds while you conjure a disturbing memory from your past. Soon the power of those bad memories is significantly reduced. (Read more about EMDR in Chapter 6) After four treatments Carol's IBS symptoms totally resolved.

Suppose you've turned over every rock and found no cause for your digestive troubles. Some doctors would then say, "It's all in your head" and there may be some truth to that—but not in the way it sounds. In many of the patients whose tests are negative, I find a past trauma at the root of their problem. My GI colleagues confirm this trend. One multicenter study of gastroenterology patients found that of those with IBS, an astounding 44% reported a past history of sexual abuse.[12]

A study from the Mayo Clinic confirmed that non-sexual traumas also contribute to IBS, finding that IBS patients are more likely than the rest of the population to have lived through physical or mental abuse, a natural disaster, a house fire, a car accident, or other trauma.[13] Any emotional episode can temporarily upset someone's intestines, but what's the link between trauma and IBS? That's not clear. It could be that trauma changes signals from the brain which control nerves in the gut. Or it may sensitize the brain and the gut in a way that leads to IBS. People with IBS may also be extra-sensitive to the normal stretching of the bowel which happens with gas and bowel movements.

If symptoms persist or I cannot find any other reason for IBS, I often prescribe acupuncture or hypnosis. The effectiveness of acupuncture for IBS patients has been studied but the results are inconclusive; some have found it helps, and others have discovered no effect. Many of my patients have experienced relief, so I regularly recommend this therapy.[14]

The studies of hypnosis for IBS have been more positive. A review of 14 studies concluded hypnosis is quite effective in resolving the symptoms of IBS.[15]

IBS symptoms are variable and can be treated in a multitude of ways. Most of my patients can resolve their symptoms through diet and alternative therapies. The key is to get to the bottom (pardon the pun) of what's going on and find the appropriate treatment.

Trust Your Gut and Take Care of It

No one argues against eating a healthy diet, but the benefits go beyond what we have traditionally believed. This was shown when one of my patients finally took my advice. What happened was amazing.

Georgia was a 70-year-old-woman I had been treating for years. She suffered from fibromyalgia, depression, and weight gain. Every time I saw her, we discussed diet and exercise and their importance in her ability to feel better. She had a tough time adhering to either.

She moved out of town and I did not see her for three years. In 2020, she came to see me for a complete exam. She had lost ten pounds, her depression was gone, and so was her fibromyalgia. What had she done?

When she moved, she followed my advice, adopted a Mediterranean-style diet, and joined a gym. She was able to get rid of her excess weight and keep it off and she started feeling happy and no longer suffered from pain.

I knew the Mediterranean diet was a good one based on epidemiologic studies.[16] After Georgia came to see me, I began to wonder why the diet worked so well, which led me to an interesting discovery. One of the main reasons the diet is successful is because it fosters healthy gut bacteria that line your intestines and help in the process of digestion. The population of gut bacteria, also known as the microbiome, is now considered an organ unto itself. The microbiome influences behavior, the immune system, cancer, heart disease risk, brain development, metabolism, and obesity, in addition to overall inflammation.[17] When Georgia started eating healthy, she improved her microbiome and reduced her inflammation, thus eliminating her pain.

Many studies show that those eating the traditional, high fat, low fiber, Western diet have disrupted gut flora. The bacteria in the gut are essential for normal metabolism. They digest food and help to produce energy, vitamins, and essential nutrients. If they are disrupted, the mucosa, the protective barrier of the intestine, can break down. This increases the intestines' permeability and allows bacteria and toxins to leak out. One of these bacteria-derived toxins is a part of the cell wall known as lipopolysaccharide or LPS. This can trigger an inflammatory response and can lead to depression. This effect has been illustrated in animal models where given LPS, the animal then exhibits depression. The induced depression is reversed by antidepressants. Equally fascinating is that in addition to the depressive response, there may be an autoimmune response to serotonin (our feel-good hormone) that is associated with fatigue.[18]

The high-fat diet increases the likelihood of increased intestinal permeability, also known as "leaky gut." The strongest influence on microbial behavior is a long-term, habitual diet. When people eat a plant-based diet rich in vegetables, fruits, and fermented food, the intestinal wall heals, there is no more leakage of LPS, and their inflammation is reduced. The College of William and Mary conducted a psychological study of students who scored high on the anxiety and neuroticism scale.[19] They discovered that students who regularly ate fermented foods showed no signs of anxious behavior. This demonstrates that the gut microbiome is at least partially responsible for anxiety.

Studies have found animals put in situations that piqued their anxiety were less likely to be anxious if they had healthy gut flora. Those with unhealthy flora suffered extreme stress. One study linked it to fat mice. Scientists painted skinny, anxious mouse poop on their front legs. The fat mice licked it off, essentially doing a fecal transplant on themselves. As a result, the fat mice lost weight and became anxious.[20] There have also been many studies showing lean mice become obese when bacteria from obese human individuals are transplanted into their gut. An experiment was performed on mice genetically predisposed to becoming fat. They were housed in the same cage with thin mice. Mice eat each other's poop (just a disgusting mouse fact). When the mice genetically programmed to be fat ate the poop of the thin mice, they did not get fat! They had done a successful stool transplant on themselves. Healthy bacteria were restored in their gut, keeping them from getting fat and preventing them from following their genes.[21]

The gut-brain connection is now widely studied, and we still have much to learn. It is entirely possible that in the future we will be treating obesity, behavioral, and mood disorders with probiotics and perhaps fecal transplants. In the meantime, improve your mood and overall well-being by boosting your good bacteria and giving them an environment where they can thrive and survive.

Prebiotics, Probiotics, And The Microbiome

You can do this by eating a healthy, clean diet rich in prebiotics that fertilize the flora. Foods that help include asparagus, beans, artichokes, garlic, root vegetables, and other foods high in fiber. In addition, fermented foods are a natural source of probiotics. Probiotics are *organisms* or *bacteria*. These include yogurt, kefir, kimchi, and sauerkraut. Avoiding antibiotics and food treated with antibiotics is also important. Antibiotics kill and alter gut bacteria, upsetting the balance of the microbiome.

You can also take probiotics in pill, liquid, powder—and even a vaginal suppository form. There are a vast number of brands and types from which to choose. Look for the type of bacteria they contain. The best probiotics have multiple types and large numbers. I most often recommend VSL#3, taken twice daily. This is a medical-grade probiotic that contains eight strains in amounts from 112.5 billion to 900 billion. The strains are:

- Bifidobacterium longum
- Bifidobacterium infantis
- Lactobacillus acidophilus
- Lactobacillus plantarum
- Lactobacillus paracasei
- Lactobacillus bulgaricus
- Streptococcus thermophilus

It is key that you know how to store the probiotics. Some, such as VSL#3, need to be refrigerated. If they are not stored properly, they will die, and you will have an expensive bunch of dead organisms that won't do you any good. Of course, if you do not change unhealthy eating habits, the probiotics won't help anyway. They need to enter an environment that helps them live and multiply for their benefit.

Exercise Will Boost Your Bacteria

Of the myriad benefits of exercise, and one which is seldom noted is that it is a natural and effective way to boost your good bacteria and keep them diversified.[22] It is something you can do every day. Exercise is an excellent way to keep the microbiome healthy. There are some promising results in athletes showing this phenomenon. Forty professional rugby players in Ireland were studied and compared to normal-weight and overweight non-athletes. The athletes had a greater diversity of bacteria and healthier guts than the non-athletes. Of course, the athletes ate a more nutritious, high-protein diet, which may explain some of the results. The next logical question: what would be seen in non-athlete exercisers compared to those who do not exercise? Fortunately, a recent study arrived at an answer.

This study looked at 104 men and women between 18 and 45. Researchers compared sedentary people to those who exercised on average three to five hours a week. In those who exercised, there was a four-fold increase in good bacteria, which boosts the immune system. These findings were more pronounced in women.[23]

How Does Exercise Do This?

Exercise increases the release of anti-inflammatory chemicals known as cytokines and myokines. It also increases the production of short-chain fatty acids that enhance bacteria that produce butyrate. Butyrate reduces the risk of colon cancer and reduces the release of the inflammatory LPS, which I mentioned earlier. It also boosts immunity by inducing the production of special regulatory T cells in the gut.[24]

Can Exercise Override Unhealthy Eating?

There is hope that it may be possible to override an occasional dietary splurge by maintaining a healthy exercise regimen. A study found that when mice exercised, they still had healthy guts despite a high-fat diet.[25] Studies in humans are pending.

A Real Killer...

One food you think might be healthy can be deadly to your gut bacteria: artificial sweeteners. The original sweetener known as saccharin was discovered completely by accident in 1879 when a chemistry research assistant at Johns Hopkins Hospital was working on a food preservative. He forgot to wash his hands before lunch and noticed the sweet taste left on the finger food he was eating. He realized he was onto something. The story (as gross as it sounds) is that he went back to his lab and tasted everything to find out where the sweetness came from. He found out that it was benzoic sulfimide, a coal tar derivative that tastes 300 times sweeter than sugar. He named this new compound after the Latin word *Saccharum*, which means sugar.[26]

Since then, many new sweeteners have been introduced to the market, often with much press and fanfare. Each of these chemicals has been heralded as nothing short of a miracle: your food and drinks are sweet and tasty with no increase in calories! What an easy way to lose weight and keep blood sugars low! Some doctors and dietitians even recommend them. The catch? Sadly, there *is* a little catch: they do not have the desired effect. Ironically, they increase glucose intolerance by altering the bacteria and doing the opposite of what they were designed to do! They *actually cause weight gain* and raise blood sugar.[27]

An extensive study was conducted in France which included over 103,000 people. Those involved in the study were, on average, 42 years old. 79.8% were women. They were followed for over 10 years, and information regarding their food and beverage consumption was collected. They used food logs accompanied by photos. They reported their artificial sweetener consumption. Thirty-seven percent used artificial sweeteners, consuming an average of 42.5 mg per day. Many included aspartame, Ace K, sucralose, cyclamates, saccharin, and steviol. The researchers collected health information and compared the number of cardiovascular events in those who consumed artificial sweeteners to those who did not. Those who were high consumers had an increased risk of cardiac events compared to those who were not. Three sweeteners were the worst; aspartame increases the risk of cerebrovascular events such as strokes, and Ace K and sucralose increase the risk of heart disease.[28] Sorry to be a buzzkill for all you diet soda drinkers. Occasional use will probably not increase your risk. However, chronic use may be a killer. Something you consume, thinking you are doing something good for your health, may do the opposite.

Inflammation is at the root of the problem with artificial sweeteners. There are other issues at play as well. What is the cause of inflammation at the microbial level?

Inflammation and the Gut

Microbes in the gut are essential for digestion. Some produce specific enzymes that help ferment nutrients to be absorbed. This includes short-chain fatty acids that have an anti-inflammatory effect. Butyrate is one of the primary short-chain fatty acids produced by exercise and various microbes.

The enzymes also release lipopolysaccharides, cell capsule carbohydrates, and endotoxins that can be released and affect the integrity of the gut wall, produce vitamins, and cause immune reactions. They can also affect how drugs are metabolized.

It is this contact with the immune system that is responsible for either *causing* or *preventing* inflammation. Bacteria can turn on regulatory cells eliciting an anti-inflammatory response or increasing the intestines' permeability and promoting a "leaky gut." Metabolites can leak into the blood, triggering a host of inflammatory responses. When cells in the gut lining deliver bacterial metabolites to immune cells, they promote inflammation locally and systemically, which is how chronic inflammation ensues. This inflammation promotes inflammatory bowel disease, diabetes, obesity, and cardiovascular disease.[29]

This provides a compelling argument for having a healthy gut microbiome. Eating a healthy diet and exercising consistently will help. Much more is being discovered regarding the science of inflammation and the microbiome. We know some, but there is so much left to learn. At least we do know what comprises a healthy lifestyle. Until the magic cocktail for gut health is invented (which I doubt will ever happen), I suggest you do the most you can to have a healthy gut and prevent disease.

• • •

Be your best partner in health.[30]

• • •

THE WRAP UP FOR GUT 101

Become a Good Partner to Yourself

You can be a great partner in your gut health if you are honest with yourself and your provider. In my experience as a wife, mother, and patient, we fool ourselves. When it comes to the gut and eating clean to feel good, we can be really good at first. But we often backslide, thinking that the short time of healthy eating will make up for indiscretions that follow.

Every little bite counts. After a while, there is a tendency to do "little cheats," but a little candy here and a little processed meat there will lead you right back to where you started.

A diet rich in primarily plant-based whole foods is optimal. The Mediterranean diet is delicious and promotes a healthy gut. A diet filled with processed meats, sugar, and highly processed foods can be destructive to the gut, and I recommend avoiding it.

• • •

When it comes to a healthy microbiome,

it is all about what you eat!

• • •

I recommended a diet known as the specific carbohydrate diet to a patient with Crohn's disease. It is a whole-food diet that restricts eating certain grains, sugar, and processed foods. She was motivated to try it to avoid medication to treat her disease. She had developed fistulas in her colon connected to the outside of her body. After following the diet they healed, and so did her Crohn's colitis. Unfortunately, she was unable to maintain the diet and relapsed. The little cheats got her. So, If you want to go the natural route, you must stick to it. The gut is quite sensitive, and it doesn't take long with an unhealthy diet to undo all the good you do eating well. On the other hand, you can see positive change relatively quickly when you adopt a healthy eating plan. Try it! You will like it. If you backslide, as many of us do, don't give up. Start again.

My patient's GI doctor started her on a medication that is helping her. If your doctor has recommendations, you need to follow them.

Partner with Your Doctor

- What you eat is essential for gut health. If you are having issues, ask your provider to help you find the best diet for you. This includes a simple blood test for celiac and food allergies and breath tests to tell you about lactose and fructose intolerance and bacterial overgrowth.

- And, if all tests are negative, a colonoscopy or upper endoscopy may be in order.

- If you have specific intolerances, avoid foods such as lactose and fructose.

PART TWO

STAY ALIVE AND THRIVE

When it comes to your health, are you where you want to be? What if your present-day self could communicate with your younger self? What would you tell her?

To My Younger Self, Here Is What I Would Have Said:

Keep exercising even when you're focused on studying and maintaining a social life. All-nighters may help you get things done to some degree, but you will be far more productive after a good night's sleep. (I never would have believed that one!) If you keep meditating, your brain will be more advanced when you get older.

And, never stop dancing. If you keep it going, you will be amazing when you get to be in your 60s! Stick with the music you love and expand your taste and horizons. Music will save your soul. Dancing to it will save your brain and your body.

Ditch the "fragels" (fried bagels that taste like donuts made at the Bagel Factory in Ann Arbor, Michigan) and all the pizza you indulge in, and eat a healthy, plant-based, whole foods diet now! I guarantee your recurrent mononucleosis symptoms will disappear. Keep having lots of sex; it is good for you. (I would have believed that one!) You will not regret it later, and you will improve your longevity and all your bodily functions.

Back to Reality

Of course, this is a fantasy, and I can't go back. However, what I did do was figure things out along the way—like getting the mono symptoms to go away and that having sex is good for me. I realized that red meat and processed foods were not healthy. I found the Mediterranean diet, which is tasty and something I can do for life. I realized that exercise is a must, and I found that dancing for me is fun and works to keep me fit. I also discovered music. It soothes me and picks me up when I am down and/or upset.

When it comes to my brain, meditation has rewired and changed me for the better. I sleep well, my memory is intact, and I feel happier and healthier. I keep learning by reading to keep up with medical literature and current events and, of course, reading spy thrillers, murder mysteries, and the occasional trashy romance novel. (As a side note, books boost your brain power whether you read them or listen to them.[1])

I have not had a problem with depression, but adding certain vitamins to my regimen has made me even happier. I have found that exercise and eating cleanly do that as well. When I occasionally cheat on my usual diet—I am human, you know!—I feel sluggish and note considerable brain fog. More proof to myself that I need to stay on a set *path to wellness.*

I keep the quotes of two of my favorite men in history (Andy Rooney and Mickey Mantle)

in the back of my mind:

Andy Rooney said,

"It's paradoxical that the idea of living a long life appeals to everyone, but the idea of getting old appeals to no one."

And Mickey Mantle said,

"If I knew I was going to live this long, I would have taken better care of myself."

Very wise men (with great points) indeed!

Life isn't just about being alive; it's about thriving and feeling great. It doesn't have to take much, at least to begin with. Once you make even one small change you will notice how much better you feel. You will want to make even more changes when you see how good you feel and connect it to that change. One good effort usually pays off double and sometimes triple—and this is especially true when it comes to your brain!

CHAPTER FOUR

BOOST YOUR BRAIN

DID YOU KNOW?

- To a certain extent **you can protect your brain** by having a healthy gut and heart.

- **You can increase your IQ** through meditation.

- **You can still learn and expand your mind** regardless of how old you are.

- **You may be able to sync** up your thoughts with others.

- **If you have an illness** such as Parkinson's, there is a way to bypass the damage done by the disease and improve your movement.

- **Sleep** is essential for a boosted brain.

- **Even if someone develops Alzheimer's disease**, they can still remember music.

We are all born with a certain amount of brain power, or intelligence, which includes the ability to reason, plan, solve problems and understand complex ideas. This compilation of qualities is often referred to as a person's intelligence quotient, or IQ, which is determined by a combination of genetics and environmental factors.[1]

There are some geniuses, but most of us "mere mortals" are not. Regardless of what we are given, there are ways to maintain and even boost our brain power throughout our lives. Of course, it takes work. All those extra brain points don't arrive out of nowhere. Boosting your brain power takes intentional effort and, for many of us, new habits. Furthermore, we must use it or lose it. In my opinion, most of the work is fun.

When it comes to increasing your brain's potential, you have more control than you realize. In this chapter, I will dig into these opportunities and provide you with new brain-boosting super-power. Together, we will look into how you can meditate and increase your IQ points, use music to calm your brain and soul, and establish a pattern of lifelong learning to continually grow more neural networks for the rest of your days. This will make life so much more fun and fulfilling.

It Is Never Too Late

Many people feel doomed to lose their brains as they age. Shrinkage of brain tissue *can* happen, and hardening of the arteries that occurs with aging *can* affect the brain's overall function because, as you know, the brain needs adequate blood and oxygen for nourishment. If it is lacking, brain tissue suffers. However, there are ways to prevent shrinkage and ways to compensate for the effects of aging. This is why I say that you can improve brain function regardless of when you start! Here are some examples:

A survey of people over 40 found that 50% do not learn something new each week. This contrasts with children and young people, who are constantly learning.[2]

If older adults acted like children when learning new things, their learning would skyrocket. Some things may be harder to grasp, but they will still change. It just takes a little longer. And this is where aging has an advantage.

One study observed that adults between 58 and 86 who took between three and five new classes for three months increased their mental abilities to the level of people 30 years younger after only a month and a half.[3]

Older people use more of their brain for certain tasks, so it is really working better. In studies of young and old adults, the younger people used their left brain for short-term memory tasks, and the older adults used both hemispheres. They could compensate this way for memory losses that occur with age. For spatial memory, younger adults showed mostly right brain activity and, again, older adults used both hemispheres to compensate for losses in the aging process.

Older people make better choices. Lower levels of testosterone in older men and women mean they have better impulse control, and mood swings are less likely when making decisions. There is a connection between impulse control and aging. Studies show a positive association between low testosterone levels and risk-seeking behaviors in economic decision-making. Socially, higher levels of testosterone are associated with being more aggressive and exhibiting more dominant behavior.

Older individuals tend to have a more extensive vocabulary, are better at problem-solving due to experience, and have better visual-spatial skills. Studies show that although social cognition may be limited as we age, it is counterbalanced by increased social expertise accumulated over a lifetime. In familiar situations, middle-aged and older adults make more accurate interpretations of the behaviors of others when compared to young adults, and their prior knowledge and experience make them more efficient in decision-making.

Older adults are usually better at basic math and can tune out negative emotions. Aging has a positive impact on mathematical ability and numerical processing. In studies, older participants earned higher mathematical achievement scores than younger participants. It appears that a lifetime of exposure to numbers leads to better mathematical achievements.

The amygdala, the part of the brain responsible for memory and emotion, is less responsive to negative situations. And older adults feel more content and accepting. In addition, oxytocin secreted by the hypothalamus, which has reciprocal connections to the amygdala, increases as we age. This is a good thing. It is associated with life satisfaction and prosocial behaviors. That may explain why we become more generous as we age.

Of course, all the above benefits are only there if our brains are healthy. Knowing this should inspire us to keep learning and building our strengths. Add healthy eating and exercise, and you have hit the brain-boosting trifecta!

• • •

Of course, *there is something more you can do.*[3]

• • •

Expand Your Mind

I have meditated on and off for four decades. It has been more "on" in the last twenty years. I meditate twice daily and often more if I have time or feel stressed. At first, it was tough to sit and focus, but now I see meditation as an oasis and find that if I forget to do it, I feel its absence. I started in college with transcendental meditation which involves focusing on a word known as a mantra and concentrating on the breath. It calmed my mind and made studying much less stressful and more productive.

Another form of meditation I enjoy is walking in nature. It is a straightforward form. I just focus on the view and the sounds, which is relaxing. Sometimes I go out to a local stable where there is a horse I groom. I learned about this from the horse experience I wrote about earlier in this book. I know it may sound weird, but the horse and I have a connection, and we meditate together as I brush her coat.

The type of meditation I do most of the time centers on visualizing light. Again, it calms me and allows me to focus more easily. I have mastered doing it anywhere or anytime. It is my go-to meditation these days. However, there are so many other ways to meditate. One of the more popular forms of meditation is:

Mindfulness Meditation

The term "mindfulness" was coined by the scientist Dr. Jon Kabat-Zinn in 1979. He described it as the awareness that comes from paying attention with purpose in the present moment and doing it without judgment. By being in the moment and concentrating on the breath, thoughts float by, producing a relaxation response and calming the mind. Mindfulness meditation helps decrease high blood pressure and improves depression.[4]

You can find many other forms of meditation online or on streaming devices. The most effective type of meditation is the one you want to do regularly and that helps quiet your mind and relax your body. The long-term positive results are substantial; the positive effect on the brain improves focus and cognition and reduces the risk of dementia. It also increases our capacity for happiness. This has been documented by MRI.[5]

A famous scientist/monk named Matthieu Ricard, termed the happiest man on earth, has been a lifelong meditator. MRI scans documented his famously huge capacity for joy as a result of meditation. Scans of his brain show excessive activity in the brain's left prefrontal cortex compared to the right. This is where happiness and joy reside.[6]

There is a theory that each person has a unique happiness set point. This is a relatively stable level. It can be decreased by traumatic life events. Fortunately, it can be increased by, you guessed it, meditation. Consistent meditation can thicken a few areas of the brain that increase your ability to cope with difficult situations. It quiets worry and increases the size of the areas for joy and pleasure, which was evidenced by examining the brain of Mr. Ricard. MRI studies of meditators have found that their amygdalas have shrunk. This is the area of the brain responsible for fear and anxiety. So, meditation decreases the worry areas and expands the areas for joy. What about one of the impediments to happiness, the overall reaction to stress marked by rising cortisol levels?[7]

A study of thirty medical students found that their cortisol levels dropped significantly after just four days of meditating for twenty minutes each day. Meditation gave them a deep sense of calm and serenity, the road to happiness.[8] These meditation studies have shown the wonderful capacity for brain neuroplasticity. There is even more evidence.

Meditation Can Improve Your Brain's Health

The benefits of meditation were seen when observing the physical structure of the brain. A study at UCLA in 2009 used MRI scans to examine the brains of long-time meditators.[9] Researchers found that the meditators' brains were larger than their non-meditating comparison group. It also affects gray matter, which is where information is processed. It is dense with nerve cells and directs sensory and motor stimuli to nerve cells in the central nervous system. More gray matter means better information processing. It gets its name due to its pinkish-gray color. According to recent studies, older people who meditate regularly do not lose gray matter as fast as non-meditators. Meditators' brains have thicker tissue in the prefrontal cortex, where we find our attention and control. The thicker, the better!

Since most of us worry about losing our minds, meditation is a safe and easy way for that NOT to happen. It will keep you from losing brain power and help you build your brain in areas that promote focus, joy, and happiness.[10]

Other studies have discovered that meditation not only improves focus; it also helps people to deal with stress. The medical student study I mentioned earlier showed that after four days of mindfulness meditation for twenty minutes daily, subjects significantly improved memory and cognition in addition to lowering their cortisol levels. Compared to non-meditators, those who meditated scored as much as ten times higher on working memory tasks. These tasks include following directions, doing mental arithmetic, and taking notes in class. Meditation improves memory and expands your brain, but can it improve your IQ? Possibly! Read on.[11]

Meditation Can Raise Your IQ

Meditation may even make us smarter. A study using brainwave training, a form of meditation, was reported in 2000. It was a case of 8-year-old identical twins with developmental delays. They were treated with twenty, thirty-minute sessions of brainwave training over twelve weeks. It increased their IQ scores by an average of 22 to 23 points. Five years later, the findings persisted. Thus far these results have all been confirmed by studying children with developmental issues.[12] Can this be extrapolated to adults and children without developmental issues? Time will tell.

What Is This Type of Meditation?

By applying electrodes to the scalp and monitoring brainwave activity, a computer shows the ebb and flow of activity and presents it to the participant. It is displayed as a video game. The game shapes brain activity to bring out positive brain waves. As the participant gets better at the game, their brainwaves and IQ improve. I tried this once to get a feel for neurofeedback. It was fun. Had I known about the IQ piece, I might have kept doing it!

But How Can Meditation Achieve These Kinds of Results?

Deep meditation slows down brain activity. Once it is slowed down, the brain rests and can improve and reorganize itself. Sort of like the body in general.[13]

To understand this, I'll explain brain waves. As you know, there are oscillating electrical voltages in the brain. They move up and down. There are five types of brain waves. I will list them from fast to slow.

- Gamma waves (35Hz) occur with concentration.

- Beta waves (12-35 Hz) occur with external attention and relaxation.

- Alpha waves (8-12 Hz) happen when you are very relaxed and have passive attention.

- Theta waves (4-8 Hz) happen with deep relaxation and inner focus and sleep.
- AND delta (0.5-4 Hz) is where your brainwaves are when you sleep.

The slower they go, the more relaxed your brain becomes. The reorganization can occur due to the lower frequency brain waves, particularly delta and theta waves generated by the meditative activity. In this state, it has time to think and repair! As a result of meditation, the brain has increased neuroplasticity, and that is how it moves functions from a damaged area of the brain to undamaged areas and actually changes the physical structure as a result of learning. I stated that delta and theta waves are more typically associated with sleep. As we'll discuss, sleep is critical to various brain functions, including memory formation, improving judgment, and reducing stress. In a way, meditation brings some beneficial functions normally found in sleep to our waking world. When you can control these various brain waves, it is amazing what you can do. It is going to seem like science fiction, but it is a real phenomenon.[14]

• • •

Don't worry, Be Happy!

• • •

Expand Your Mind, Sync Your Brain

Dr. Jaogo Grinberg-Zylerbaum is a neuroscientist who worked with shamans and others in Mexico collecting electroencephalographs, otherwise known as EEG or brainwave information relevant to learning, memory, perception, and biopsychology. In plain language, he was studying mental telepathy. Can we communicate with others without using words but using brain waves?

In 1987, he experimented by having two people meditate together for 20 minutes. He then separated them into two different rooms, both shielded from electromagnetic energies so there was no way to communicate with hidden devices.

One person was presented with random flashes of light. The other person sitting in a different room was hooked to an EEG machine. The second subject's EEG readings sometimes showed similar shock responses, which were accurately timed to the first subject's exposure to the flashing light. This seeming synchronization happened 25% of the time. The control group had no such responses as the second subject.

He did more than fifty experiments over five years, concluding that there was a possibility that, under certain conditions, two separated subjects might have correlated brain activity, a mental connection, aka mental telepathy. Though his findings were heavily criticized, Grinberg-Zylberbaum's findings have been independently verified by several other researchers.[15]

As a side note, in 1994, Dr. Jacobo Grinberg- Zylberbaum disappeared under mysterious circumstances. Why? No one is sure. His exploration of psychophysiology outside of traditional science may have had something to do with it. I hope he is enjoying himself in a think tank somewhere on a peaceful mountaintop.

His findings lead us to the intriguing possibility that meditation may help us do more than find ourselves but also potentially connect to others. Perhaps there can be such a thing as a local or even a global consciousness with which we can commune. If this is a real phenomenon, just think what positive thoughts can do when sent out into the world! It sounds like the stuff of pure science fiction, but the possibilities for future research are fascinating.

Meditation is an ancient practice for a reason. As an adjunct to a healthy lifestyle, it has a range of benefits for both health and happiness. It's free and easy to learn, there's definitely no risk but significant benefits to your health and, for many people, its impact can be profound.

A patient of mine had resistant high blood pressure which stayed high no matter what medications were added to his regimen. Being uptight by nature, his blood pressure totally stressed him out. He was checking it five to six times a day. I suggested he start meditating. He was skeptical but studiously began mindfulness meditation. It helped that the scientist Jon Kabat-Zinn was my backup authority. He followed the recommendations in the program that Kabat-Zinn outlined and, by a miracle of miracles, the patient's blood pressure came down. This was much to the amazement of the patient and the specialist treating his blood pressure! More proof that our brains can expand and do incredible things. Learning is another one of those mind-expanding activities that may be more difficult as we age but well worth the effort.

Lifelong Learning

If, at first, you don't succeed, try try again is more than an adage promoting tenacity and practice. It's excellent advice for keeping your brain healthy! The more you learn or try to learn, the better your brain will be able to understand.

This has been shown repeatedly by studies done with the Osher Lifelong Learning Institute (OLLI).[16] The institute sponsors educational programs nationwide for adults over 50 to increase cognitive and social engagement. Courses on a variety of topics are offered.

One of the oldest programs was started in Delaware in 1980. From 2000 to 2019, between 2100 and 2400 OLLI members took classes every semester in Wilmington. There were 65 courses and 40 extracurricular activities offered for 14-week semesters. The program is designed to stimulate the brain and encourage socialization. History is one of the participants' favorite topics. Courses in performing arts, including music, band, chorus, and choirs, stimulate multiple areas of the brain. There are foreign language studies, exercise classes, and even lectures on travel.

A study was performed by the music committee to find out how the participants benefited from their experience. Seventy-two members were included who listed the three most important benefits. Eight categories were identified.

Number one was the opportunity to sing with peers (72%), followed by friendship (64%), learning new music (53%), professional leadership (43%), singing beautiful music (38%), feeling happy (34%), and enjoying the performance (30%).

Interestingly, having improved health from singing was important but last on the list at 23%. Obviously, enjoyment kept these participants coming back!

The average length of participation in these programs is 8.1 years. Participants enjoy the engagement mentally and socially and reduce their risk for cognitive decline. It is great to know that these programs are available nationwide and open to those 50 and older. This is a wonderful way to maintain brain power and a fun way to use it, so you don't lose it![17]

Another way to help your brain with regards to learning and just about everything else is to get adequate sleep.

Sleep to Power Your Brain

What is amazing about sleep is that we are still somewhat "in the dark" with regards to why we need it. We spend roughly a third of our lives sleeping. We know that rest is essential for growth, weight control, and overall good physical health, and it is necessary for good mental health.

A poor night's sleep can ruin your day. It turns out that the parts of the brain that rule emotions (specifically the amygdala) can override our more logical part of the brain (the prefrontal cortex) when we are sleep deprived. That helps to explain why many are so emotional when exhausted and why chronic sleep deprivation can lead to depression and anxiety.[18]

On the other hand, a good night's sleep can make you feel like a million bucks! You will be focused and energetic. Some people act as if sleep is mere self-indulgence and discount it, so it is not a priority. Unfortunately for them, it is an unhealthy approach. It is key to our health and well-being.

What Is Happening?

There is a neurochemical produced in the brain known as adenosine. It governs our sleep-wake cycle. It builds up during the day and is cleaned away when we sleep. If we do not get adequate sleep, it sticks around and makes us feel foggy and groggy. If you nap, that can help clear some of it, but a good night's sleep is really what you need.

People who get less than 8 hours of sleep often have impaired memory and cognition. They are more prone to inattention and are more likely to have car accidents due to losing focus. Tired drivers are estimated to be responsible for 50,000 injuries and 800 fatalities a year in the US alone. Actually, AAA estimates there are 328,000 crashes annually due to drowsy drivers.[19]

Lack of sleep is also responsible for increased risks of heart disease, high blood pressure, diabetes, stroke, obesity, and depression. It also increases the risk of injury in adults, teens, and children. As if this isn't scary enough, sleep deficiency has also played a role in human mistakes linked to tragic accidents, such as nuclear reactor meltdowns, the grounding of large ships, and plane crashes.[20]

Seven to eight hours is ideal for those over 65. It turns out that about a third of Americans sleep less than 6 hours a night. Fifty to seventy million people in the US suffer from chronic sleep disorders; we are not alone. Up to 30% of people around the world suffer from insomnia.[21]

• • •

So many things going on at night

while your eyes are closed!

• • •

– SLEEP 101 –

The best place to start is by getting some information. Are you getting enough sleep, and are you getting enough good sleep? Sleep is made up of a variety of cycles. We know about REM sleep. It is talked and written about all the time. It is where we dream.[22]

In addition to REM, there is non-REM sleep.

There are five stages of sleep: wake, N1, N2, N3, and REM. The N stages refer to non-rapid eye movement sleep, and with each increasing number, we go deeper into sleep. Each stage is important. Most of the time we sleep (75%) is spent in NREM. The N2 is the majority of time spent in this stage. A healthy night's sleep consists of 4 to 5 cycles. The cycle order is N1, N2, N3, N2, and REM. Each cycle takes 90 to 110 minutes.

The first REM period is short. As the night unfolds, there are progressively longer periods of REM. Deep sleep occurs for more prolonged periods earlier in the sleep cycle and decreases over time.[23]

Why we dream is still not fully understood. It may be a way of cataloging and incorporating activities and experiences during the day. Even though we may not completely understand why we dream, we do know it is essential.

For this reason, it is important to know what interferes with REM. One of the main things is alcohol. When you drink before falling asleep, REM is disrupted. Once the alcohol wears off in the middle of the night, REM starts up again and makes up for the lost time. This often results in vivid dreams and nightmares.

Interestingly, there is something else that will disrupt it; travel. Only half our brain sleeps when we are in a in a hotel bed or an unfamiliar place. The other half is on alert. In addition to jet lag, which messes with our circadian or body rhythm, this may be another reason for not feeling as rested as usual when we are on a trip.

Deep sleep is essential so the body can release growth hormones and repair muscles, bones and tissues, and the immune system. It is also crucial for cognitive function. The brain needs it to evaluate and consolidate memories.

How much do we need? It is a percentage of the total hours we sleep. So, between 13% and 23% is the key. If we get seven hours a night, it is optimal to spend between 55 and 97 minutes each night in deep sleep.[23]

Good Sleep Starts with Good Habits!

So, how do you know you are getting enough REM and Non-REM sleep? This is not information you can intuit. Just getting the requisite number of hours may not be enough. You may need help. There are Fitbits (cost as low as $50), special mattresses ($600 to over $9000), and Oura rings ($300). They can tell if you are getting the quantity and quality of sleep you need. They monitor your movements, heart rate, respiration, and body temperature. Some even offer advice on how to achieve better sleep. I have some tips of my own for you!

Tips for a good night's sleep:

- Set a sleep schedule. Go to bed at the same time every night and wake at the same time in the morning. Want to reset your clock? Camping is an excellent way to do that. If you are like me and camping is not your favorite activity, try glamping! You go to sleep when the sun goes down and rise when it comes back up!

- Keep your room cool.

- If you can, ban screens from your bedroom.

- Use your bed only for sex and sleeping.

- If you wake up in the middle of the night, rather than toss and turn, you can get up and meditate or read or listen to a relaxing story or app until you get sleepy.

- Exercise regularly.

- Avoid alcohol 3 hours before bedtime.

- Avoid eating at least 2 hours before bedtime.

- Avoid caffeine after 2 PM.

If these tips don't help, you may have a sleeping disorder and it is time to see your doctor. You (and your doctor) may be tempted by a pill. As a physician who has been around a while, I urge patients to stay away from prescription sleep meds. They may help you sleep, but often it is not restorative sleep. (Restorative sleep being defined as sleep that includes deep sleep and REM). That is where the devices help. They can identify whether you made it into those stages or not.

Some of the scariest stories come from those who have used Ambien (Zolpidem), a common medication prescribed for sleep. I have had patients found wandering in their nightgowns at night with no idea what they are doing. Others could not figure out how they were gaining weight and found out they had been eating in the middle of the night. Others had sex and did not remember it.

There are so many creative ways to improve sleep these days. It makes sense to try them before jumping to a pill. Hypnotherapy, Cognitive Behavioral Therapy, relaxation therapy, acupuncture, and meditation are techniques proven to help with sleep issues.[24]

If you feel you need to take something, teas such as chamomile and an amino acid known as theanine can help you relax and get to sleep. Theanine comes in many forms and is safe. There are other over-the-counter natural sleep remedies available. Discussing these with your doctor before trying them is always a good idea. Some calming music, perhaps?

A Musical Rewire For The Brain

Music helps the brain by providing significant therapeutic benefits. There are a variety of ways it can do this. From infants to the elderly and to the infirm, it has a healing effect.

When It Comes to Babies…

A study published in the journal Pediatrics in 2013 found that lullabies played in the neonatal intensive care unit (NICU) soothe pre-term babies along with their parents. It improves their eating and sleeping patterns (the baby's that is) and reduces their parents' stress levels.[25]

Another study looked at 272 premature babies 32 weeks' gestation and older being cared for in mid-Atlantic NICUs. Three types of music were played: a lullaby sung by the baby's parents, an "ocean disc," and a round instrument invented by the Remo drum company that mimics sounds of the womb along with a gato box, a drum-like instrument used to simulate a heartbeat. The musical instruments played by music therapists matched the beats to the babies' breathing and heart rhythms.[26]

Interestingly, all the modalities slowed the baby's heart rate; singing seems to be the most effective for keeping the babies quiet and alert. The gato box improved their sucking behavior. The ocean disc enhanced sleep. Music has a profound effect at a deep level when you see what impact it has on babies, and it doesn't stop there!

In Children and Adults

Many current studies show the benefits of music for mental and physical health. A 2013 meta-analysis of 400 studies (combined data of multiple research studies) found that music improves immune system function and reduces stress in the body. It was also found to be more effective than prescription drugs for reducing anxiety before surgery.[27]

Both listening to and playing music increases the body's production of natural killer cells and immunoglobulin that protect the body from viral invaders. In addition, it reduces the stress hormone cortisol thus proving that the relaxation many of us experience with music has a real physiologic basis.

Canadian researchers who followed 42 children from 3 to 11 years old in an emergency room at the University of Alberta found that when the children listened to relaxing music while an IV was started, they reported less pain and noted less distress than those who did not listen to music. Those health care providers inserting the IVs found them easier to insert compared to 38% of those treating the patients who did not listen to music.[28]

Playing music for children or adults during painful procedures makes sense as an intervention. It causes no harm and has a soothing effect. Music has been particularly powerful when treating patients in palliative care (those dealing with a terminal disease).

The Infirm

A study in Singapore found that when patients took part in live music therapy sessions, they had relief from persistent pain. The patients took part in singing, instrument playing, and even songwriting as they dealt with their end-of-life issues. Engaging in music allowed them to reconnect with the healthy part of themselves despite the pain and disability created by their disease. It allowed them to truly rest.[29]

As to issues involving speech difficulties, especially in those who have experienced a brain injury or stroke, music is an invaluable tool. This has been known for quite a long time. In an article entitled, "Singing by Speechless Children" published in 1871, neurologist, Dr. John Hughlings Jackson discussed his findings, noting that when people cannot access words to speak, they can often find them by singing.[30] Music tricks the brain into finding the words they cannot access otherwise. This was played out in the media when Senator Gabby Giffords suffered a gunshot wound to her brain and could not speak. She was unable to express herself, a condition known as aphasia. After many intensive sessions, she recovered her words through song. Starting with "Happy Birthday," "American Pie," and "Brown Eyed Girl," Gabby made her way back to speaking again.[31]

That is remarkable, but as if that isn't enough, there's more! Music's greatest and most impressive impact on disease is seen with neurodegenerative disorders like multiple sclerosis, motor neuron disease, and Parkinson's disease. In Parkinson's disease, patients develop a shuffling gait and difficulty initiating movement, and some suffer freezing, where movement stops abruptly. We use external rhythmic cues for our internal timing. This involves many networks in the brain's frontal area, connected across the basal ganglia to the cerebellar motor networks. As you may recall, the basal ganglia of the brain is the diseased area in Parkinson's.

So, to help with gait in those with Parkinson's disease, it is necessary to restore the cerebral mechanisms that generate walking rhythm. The use of cues is what seems to be important for patients. Visual or auditory signals help with gait and induce redirection to neural circuits less affected by the disease. Musical cues assist with this process as patients try to match their steps to the beat and redevelop a normal gait while reducing the incidence of freezing.[32]

Studies show that internal cues in the form of singing are even more beneficial than external cueing with music for this process. In other words, energetic music with singing by the patient may provide better motor benefits than passive listening. The release of endorphins and oxytocin during singing also helps with motivation and better output for movement. Synchronizing movement with their voice appears to lead patients to greater activation of their motor networks. The same factors are at play regarding the therapeutic benefit of singing and speech. When singing, there is continuous voicing and syllable lengthening, leading to better connectedness between words. This may translate to motor impairments as well. The variability of speech and movement may be reduced for both with singing.

Music therapy has also been studied for patients with Alzheimer's disease and other forms of dementia. Patients often retain their memory for music even though they experience cognitive decline in different aspects. In the Brain chapter, I offered the example of Tony Bennett, who has the ability to remember songs despite suffering from severe Alzheimer's disease. His experience is an example of how the brain's musical networks act separately from the temporal lobe memory networks and are spared by dementia. This means that music can be a powerful cue to evoke memories that can prompt emotional responses in addition to the memory of the music. In fact, music is one of the most powerful ways to bypass the degeneration caused by dementia, trigger autobiographical memories on behalf of the sufferer, and make them feel connected with themselves and the outside world.[33]

There are many ways to supercharge and boost your brain. Meditation, music, ensuring plenty of good quality sleep, and continuing to learn throughout your life can all help keep your mind fit and happy. Your brain determines how you are uniquely *you*. We each have much to contribute. If we do not use what is available to us to maintain and increase our brain power, we will lose it. That is why it is vital to take care of your brain and realize its tremendous power. As Mary Oliver wrote, "Don't waste your one wild and precious life." Do whatever it takes to have the healthiest, boosted brain possible!

CHAPTER FIVE

LONGEVITY: AN AGE-OLD QUESTION

Aging is a given in life; an unstoppable process for all of us. But, *how we age* can vary from person to person. Genetics is a factor and largely out of our control, but our lifestyle choices heavily influence how we age. As an example, smoking is an age accelerator.[1] Smokers develop premature wrinkling and aging of the skin due to narrowing of the blood vessels, thus depriving the skin of the nutrients it needs. In addition, the acceleration of blood vessel narrowing causes the entire body to age more quickly.

Healthy aging takes work just like everything else, but it is worth it! Although the COVID pandemic has decreased the average life span of adults in the US, it's still possible for many of us over 60 to live to see our one-hundredth birthday. But what is the point unless our quality of life is good? In this chapter, we explore the theories on how we age and you will discover why some people can live into their 100s healthily. You will learn what you can do to slow the aging process and even turn back the clock by making healthy lifestyle choices. The researchers at Stanford are not only helping to define the aging process but are finding ways to slow it down or even reverse it to some degree so we can have a good quality of life as we get older. To do this, we need to understand how aging happens.

To help with this, the Stanford Center on Longevity has launched an initiative known as The New Map of Life,[2] designed to meet the challenge of those who live longer. For starters, they have found a protein level in people's blood that can predict their age. They have a physiological clock that looks at the level of 373 circulating proteins in the blood. The levels of these proteins may be responsible for aging.

A study of 4263 people between 18 and 95 found that physiologic aging does not occur at a regular pace but is more of a jerky process. They found three inflection points in our life cycle when the proteins change: 34, 60, and 78. The levels of many proteins will remain steady for a while and then undergo an upward or downward shift at some point. These shifts happen in young adulthood, late middle age, and old age. Using this model, the researchers could predict individuals' ages within a range of 3 years most of the time. If the expected age was substantially lower than the actual age, the reason was that the person was remarkably healthy.[3]

The samples from these studies came from the Longevity study, a registry of exceptionally long-lived Ashkenazi Jews, many of whom live to the age of 95. Of the 3000 proteins studied, they found 1379 proteins of varying levels. When they reduced them to 373, they could predict ages with accuracy. A good predictor of a younger-than-predicted age was hand-grip strength and cognitive function. The study also showed that men and women age differently. Of the proteins analyzed, 895 were more predictive for one sex than the other. It's not surprising that men and women age differently![4]

This is all well and good. We age at different rates depending on how healthy we are. How does that happen? Perhaps, the theories on aging will explain this. This might help you understand the more profound "molecular reasons" to make healthy lifestyle choices.

Ok, So How Do We Age Then?

Drilling down, how does aging happen, and is age just a number? Not always. The younger-than-stated age group has shown that. While there are many theories, and scientists are very busy figuring out the answer, we still don't know exactly why our bodies age. One view is that our genes determine how long we live. Another is that our DNA becomes damaged over time; it can't recover, ultimately leading to our demise. Let me explain a little about DNA and how it is put together.

We have 23 chromosomes that contain our genes. They carry information, like a map, on how each of us is put together. They dictate our eye color, skin color, and even our hair color. They literally make us who we are. Every cell in the human body contains 23 pairs of such chromosomes.[5]

On the end of each chromosome are telomeres made from DNA sequences and proteins. They are protective caps, just like what you see on the ends of shoelaces. As we age, they shorten. They can be replenished with an enzyme called telomerase. However, those "shoelace" tips still shrink with every cell division, so the cells will start to fade or die. We know telomere damage affects aging from studies performed on mice. Those with short telomeres live shorter lives. In humans, mutated telomerase is associated with an increased risk of cancer. The telomeres are at increased risk of damage from external stress, which might explain the differences in how individuals age.

Beyond telomeres, there is another theory that mitochondria are behind the aging process. Mitochondria are in almost every cell in the body. They energize the cells. Mitochondria have little mini-organs (organelles) residing inside them. They release energy from food. This is called cellular respiration.[6]

For this reason, mitochondria are our cells' power stations. They have their own pool of DNA, and DNA in mitochondria has more mutations than elsewhere. This is due to a lack of self-protective mechanisms and limited repair abilities, which makes them more susceptible to damage and, as a result, it makes us more vulnerable to disease. When the mitochondria produce energy, if they are not balanced, they create what we call oxidative stress, which can damage DNA and contribute to aging, cancer, and neurodegenerative diseases (to name a few).

Another fascinating theory about aging deals with the cells themselves. Scientists have discovered that the aging process causes regulators that circulate in the blood to be released. Regulators are proteins that bind to genes and regulate how they are expressed. They can turn them on or off. One of them is called growth differentiation factor 11, or GDF11, a protein that researchers have found may reverse aging, at least in mice. A paper published in 2014 states that it rejuvenates mice brains. Older mice treated with this protein had improved function and could smell odors typically only picked up by younger mice.[7] The level of GDF-11 in mice and humans decreases with age.

A group of Harvard Medical School researchers surgically joined young and old mice. (I don't even want to know how they did that!) They found that young blood restored some of the lost function of the older mice's heart, brain, and skeletal muscles, and using GDF11 alone gave the same result. The next question is, would treating humans with GDF11 do the same thing? Only time and research will tell.

These theories give hope for how we can possibly improve our chances of aging well. If we can avoid precipitating oxidative stress in our mitochondria and promote healthy telomeres by living a healthy lifestyle, it is possible to fool the Stanford folks and be younger than the age on our driver's license. This applies to brain health as well.

Aging and the Brain

Stanford scientist Katrin Andreasson, along with her colleagues, has found a critical factor in mental aging—amazingly, it has to do with our immune system.[8] Over time, for some people the immune system goes a bit haywire. It does the opposite of what is expected and causes inflammation. This inflammation is at the root of heart disease, Alzheimer's disease, cancer, and failure to thrive in general. The big question has been, which immune cells are the problem? And now these researchers think they have found them.

Myeloid cells are in the brain and circulatory system. They fight infection, clean debris such as dead cells and clumps of protein and watch for invaders such as cancer cells. But as we age, our myeloid cells get tired and slack off. They may even get confused, adopt a new agenda, and fight enemies that aren't there, hurting innocent tissues such as the brain with resulting deterioration. A different group of Stanford researchers discovered that by adjusting the immune system, they could de-age the brain. In mouse studies, blocking the signals of myeloid cells restored youthful metabolism. It also reversed the mental decline.[9]

The myeloid cells create a positive feedback loop interacting with hormones and their receptors, creating inflammation. They hoard glucose (sugar) instead of spending it. When the cells become energy depleted, they go into an inflammatory rage and hurt aging tissues. Think "hangry."

This process can be blocked using a chemical compound. By doing this, the cells can go ahead and metabolize the sugar and reverse the inflammation. In mice, this process reversed their age-related cognitive decline. Even if the compound did not get into the brain tissue, it had a positive effect. Although the compound is not toxic in mice, we do not yet know how it works in humans. Understanding the mechanism, human trials will be forthcoming. We are one step closer to reversing the brain and body aging process.

In another exciting development, Harvard researchers have found a signature of human longevity in the genes of the brain's cerebral cortex. It involves slowing down the impulses in the brain, keeping it from getting too excited. Let me explain.

Brain signals are in the form of electrical currents. (Remember, the brain can power a 25-watt bulb!) When too much activity or the neural network gets over excited, a mood change, or muscle twitching can occur.

In the Harvard study, the researchers did cellular, genetic, and molecular experiments in worms and mice with altered genes. They also looked at the brain tissue of people over 100 years old after they died. The tests found that altering neural activity could influence life span.

Tying into what the Stanford researchers found, glucose (sugar) metabolism is important in aging. That is why it is not surprising that signaling by the hormones insulin and insulin-like growth factor (IGF) influences longevity. Also, neural excitation affects longevity down this pathway. And it does it with the help of a transcription factor named REST.[10]

Transcription factors are proteins/regulators (Remember the GDF-11 story?) that switch genes on and off. It depends on *how* they are turned on and off as to their effect on an individual cell and individual people. This mechanism helps us cope with different reactions to our environment. REST can help protect the brain from the stress of damaged nerve cells, such as what happens in dementia.

REST suppresses neural activity in animal models, worms, and mammals. It does it for genes that have an essential role in the excitation of the nerves. When researchers blocked REST in testing animal models, the neural activity rose, and the life span of the animals was cut short. Boosting REST had the opposite effect; the animals lived longer.

Looking at the brains of people who lived beyond 100 years revealed higher levels of REST in their cells compared to those whose life span was between 20 and 30 years shorter. Lower neural activity does something else. It switches on a group of proteins called forkhead transcription factors.[11] These weirdly named proteins influence longevity through the same insulin and IGF signaling pathways. This human neural activity variation could be due to genetic and environmental factors. This is a reason to keep your brain as robust as possible by maintaining a healthy lifestyle, avoiding long-term stress, and exercising regularly.

To avoid deprivation of essentials necessary for the brain to prevent disease, oxygenated blood must be pumped in to nourish and keep it working. All the regulators and weird little proteins can't do their thing without a healthy heart.

The Heart and Longevity

Obviously, you need your heart to do what it does so well throughout your life and to keep you going as long as possible. We've discussed healthy eating, exercise, dealing with stress, not smoking, and maintaining normal blood pressure.

But there is another beacon worth paying attention to, your pulse.

A study was published in Sweden in 2019 where 798 men were tracked between 1993 and 2014. The men were divided into four groups based on their resting heart rates. They were as follows: 55 beats per minute (bpm) or less, 56 bpm to 65 bpm, 66 bpm to 75 bpm, and more than 75 bpm.[12]

Researchers found that resting heart rates can identify men who are likely or less likely to suffer a cardiac event. Those whose resting heart rate sits between 50 and 60 are 44% less likely to suffer heart disease before 71 than those with higher pulse rates. The data showed that every bpm increase between 50 and 60 boosts the risk of death by 3% during the next 11 years. They also found that those with a resting heart rate of 75 beats per minute or higher were twice as likely to die of heart disease within 11 years than their peers with a heart rate of 55 bpm or less.

These numbers show us why it's so essential to stay healthy and active over our entire lifetime. In general, the elevated heart rate is a red flag identifying those most likely to be inactive, stressed out, eat poorly, and/or smoke. More studies are needed. Women were not included in this but must be part of future research.

In the meantime, there is no harm in working on your fitness level and trying to lower your pulse rate by adopting healthy habits. It may help you to live a long and healthy life.

Part of "having a healthy life" means paying close attention to your gut. As you will see, it is very essential for healthy aging. Even *I* had no idea until I took a closer look.

OMG, THIS IS AMAZING!

The Gut Microbiome and Aging

Scientists know that people who live to be 100 and older are less susceptible to chronic diseases and more likely to survive infectious diseases. A 2021 study reveals that these individuals have a unique microbiome, which may be why they are protected from bacterial infections and infections that have become antibiotic-resistant.[13]

Another study looked at the genetics of the gut microbiome from more than 9000 people between the ages of 18 and 101, paying close attention to the 900 older adults in the community. Those who had a unique pattern of their GI microbiome profile tended to be healthier and live longer than their adult peers who did not. Their blood tests revealed lower LDL (harmful cholesterol) levels and higher vitamin D levels. They also found a healthy gut metabolite called tryptophan-derived-indole. This has been shown to reduce inflammation and help mice live longer.

The older human individuals with the unique microbiome walked faster and were more mobile than those with less diverse microbes. Those with a less varied microbiome were on more medications and more than twice as likely to die during the study period. The researchers surmised that the lack of diversity in their microbiome was probably due to salt, sugar, processed foods, and fatty meats which can damage any gut but particularly the aging one.

A whole food, plant-based diet rich in fruits and veggies and seeds, beans, and nuts, along with plenty of exercise, is the way to go if you want to be like the amazing seniors with a unique microbiome. My mother is one of these people. If they studied her microbiome, I am sure she would be pretty special. She has practiced all these healthy lifestyle behaviors her entire life, and it shows inside and out!

Now, you have some idea about theories of aging and how vital your brain, heart, and gut are to the process. Next, I will discuss the biological pathways to aging and how you personally can affect and possibly alter them in a good way.

The Mechanics of Aging

There is good news about the mechanics of aging, and it's fascinating stuff! Researchers have found the specific biological pathways along which we age. They are called ageotypes.[14] There are four: metabolic, immune, hepatic (liver), and nephrotic(kidney). What do they mean? People with diabetes (metabolic), when out of control with elevated Hemoglobin A1C levels (used as a marker for blood sugar levels), will age more quickly compared to those with normal blood sugar. Those with immune issues such as autoimmune disease who have elevated immune markers in their blood, such as C-reactive protein, may age more quickly than those with normal markers.

Similarly, those with liver and/or kidney disease may age more rapidly than those with normal liver and/or kidney function. They are not mutually exclusive and can compound when added (e.g., diabetes + liver disease increases aging versus diabetes alone). We have known for years that markers like high cholesterol are more common in aging populations. But what else is going on?

The ageotype researchers profiled 43 healthy men and women between the ages of 34 and 68. They took lots of blood and measurements at least five times over two years and noted that people age along different biological pathways.

As I mentioned, a single individual can have several aging processes going on at once. The good news is that if this happens, the individual can *reverse* these markers and decrease or even reverse aging. For instance, lowering Hemoglobin A1C by improving diet and exercising, and reducing inflammatory markers with diet, stress management, and exercise can do it. Interestingly, they looked at the differences in aging between healthy participants and those who were insulin resistant. Ten molecules differed significantly between them, and those markers were involved in immune function and inflammation. By modifying lifestyles and reducing sugars, the team saw aging markers decrease. This occurred not only in Hemoglobin A1C levels and inflammatory markers but also in kidney function.[14]

Modifying lifestyle and diet can decrease your markers for aging. In other words, you can lower your physiological age. Different systems age at different rates. You can improve your ageotypes by living your best life.

So how do you live your best life? For this, we need to take an epidemiologic view of aging. We don't age by biology alone; it also has to do with our behavior—and that's a good thing! It means regardless of our genetics; we can improve our life expectancy and our quality of that long life.

I Have Good News

In 1921, Lewis Terman, a psychologist at Stanford University, launched a study of more than 1500 bright children about ten years old. The study followed these children throughout their lives, studying their family histories, relationships, hobbies, pets, jobs, educational success, and many other factors. The original plan was to observe them for six months. Instead, the study continues to this day, with only 200 of his subjects still alive.[15] It has yielded some surprising findings, such as:

- Marriage is essential for men's health but not for women. Men who stayed in long-term marriages were more likely to make it past 70. Less than a third of divorced men made it beyond 70. Men who never married lived longer than divorced men, but not as long as married men. Being divorced was much less harmful to women's health. It did not affect life expectancy.

- Productivity is important. Those involved and committed to their jobs lived longer than those who were not.

- *Kids need to play.* Those who began first grade before age six were at higher risk for early mortality.

- Playing with pets is not associated with longer life.

- Combat veterans are at risk for early mortality due to unhealthy patterns rather than the trauma of combat. Those who could find meaning in the experience were more likely to find a healthy way to live.

Another landmark longevity study is the Grant Study of Harvard Alumni.[16] The research began in 1938 and examined the psychological and physical health of 268 members of Harvard classes between 1939 and 1944. Two of the distinguished members of the study were John F. Kennedy and famed newspaper editor Ben Bradlee. (As an interesting aside, Leonard Bernstein and Norman Mailer were rejected.) The study also included 456 men from inner-city Boston between 1940 and 1945 studied as controls for juvenile delinquency.

In addition to rigorous physical exams and regular checkups, the subjects answer extensive questionnaires every two years, give in-depth interviews, and submit DNA blood tests and neuroimaging. Many participants have lived into their 80s and 90s, and Harvard is now doing the Second Generation Study, learning about the children of the original participants. The participants' wives have also been asked to engage in the interview process to offer a more complete picture. Here are some of the key findings:

- Having a tough childhood significantly impacts early adulthood, but the effects of a difficult childhood fade over time.

- Those who are self-starters and get jobs as kids live longer than those who do not.

- Attending college determines lifetime success more than money or social status.

- One's situation at age 50 has more to do with health and happiness at 70 than what happened earlier in life.

- The ability to play in childhood is a better indicator of late-life happiness rather than income.

- A stable marriage is correlated to late-life happiness.

- Alcohol was a significant factor in 57% of the divorces in the Grant Study.

- Although genetics play a role, lifestyle choices significantly impact longevity and happiness.

This study confirms the value of adopting a healthy lifestyle for well-being and physical health. It's also encouraging to know one can get over a difficult childhood and still happily thrive after 50; the resilience of the human spirit—and the human body—has been proven once again!

And, as if this isn't enough evidence about healthy living leading to a long life, there are still the Blue Zones to consider.[17] The Blue Zones were so named in 2004 when Dan Buettner, along with National Geographic, explored areas around the world where people live the longest and healthiest. To qualify, longevity at a national level needed to rank among the highest in the world level based on age, sex, and life expectancies observed in censuses. Buettner identified these areas and circled them in blue, which is how the Blue Zones got their name.

These Blue Zones include Okinawa, Japan, where women live longer than any women on the planet; Sardinia, Italy, which had the highest concentrations of male centenarians; Nicoya Peninsula, Costa Rica, had the second highest concentration of male centenarians; Ikaria, Greece, which had the lowest rates of dementia in the world, and Loma Linda, California, wherein the Adventist community people lived 10 years longer than their peers in North America. These areas had nine things in common, which Buettner called the *Power 9*[17]:

- **Move**: They all move naturally throughout their lives. They garden, walk to the store, and visit their neighbors.

- **Find your purpose**: They have a sense of purpose which scientists have found adds at least 7 years to their lives.

- **De-stress**: They know how to downshift and deal with stress. Some pray, others take naps, and others take time out of the day to remember ancestors. Sardinians have a regular happy hour (and have some of the best wine on the planet!)

- **Don't stuff yourself**: They stop eating when they are 80% full. This is called Hara Hachi Bu. (My husband has not mastered this…we call him Hara Hachi Bu Bu!)

- **Feast on plants**: Their diet is primarily plant-based. They eat small servings of meat very infrequently. They eat a LOT of beans.

- **Drink in moderation**: Except for the Adventists in Loma Linda, they all drink moderately (no more than 1-2 a day) regularly. The drinkers outlive the non-drinkers.

- **Have faith**: Almost all of the centenarians belong to a faith-based community. According to research, attending faith-based services 4 times a month can add between 4 and 14 years to your life.

- **Family first**: Family comes first. They keep older parents and grandparents close. They are respected and revered.

- **Find your friends**: They have strong social networks. They have a close-knit group of friends with healthy habits. These are contagious in a beautiful way!

You can see how those around the world and here in the US can live not just a long life but a healthy and productive one. Many of the adopted habits and lifestyles are relatively easy to do. When we look at how we age, you will understand why this information is so valuable.

And One More Thing!

Longevity-focused lifestyle changes go beyond exercise and eating well. Having passionate activities can have a massive influence on well-being and aging. Adding playfulness can help, too, as an interesting study out of Pennsylvania State University showed.[18]

Researchers explored the relationship between healthy aging and playfulness—all Blue Zones have playfulness in common—and identified fifteen qualities. They were:

happy	naughty
optimistic	clowning
cheerful	teasing
joyful	creative
positive	whimsical
relaxed	funny
enthusiastic	humorous
mischievous	

They postulate that adult playfulness is essential to cognitive function and emotional growth in aging. My personal experience with this is witnessing my mother, who has all fifteen qualities and is sharp as a tack.

The exciting news is that we are coming close to explaining how each of us can live long, healthy, fulfilling lives. The key is keeping our bodies as healthy as we can—and that comes back to lifestyle choices.

Keep your diet clean with whole foods and plenty of plant-based items, including veggies, fruit, and lots of BEANS! (And I am not talking about refried.)

Find a daily way to move. Make it something you enjoy, and then you will keep doing it. Garden, take a walk in the park, or, better yet, get a dog. (Then you will have someone to make you get out and move.) Find a purpose that excites you. Spend time with your friends and family.

Here are a few more reminders you have likely already heard and hopefully you've already heeded. To preserve the skin, avoid the sun or use hats and sunscreen. To protect lung and cardiac function, do not smoke. If you smoke, quit. Exercise regularly and eat a heart-healthy diet (The Mediterranean diet discussed in Chapter 9). For a healthy gut, eat a healthy diet and do your regular screenings for colon cancer starting at age 50 or sooner, depending on your family history.

• • •

The secret to the fountain of youth

• • •

Remember: there is no magic pill to swallow or water to drink from a magic stream that will unlock your youthfulness and longevity. That's the stuff of fairy tales and deceptive advertising. *The secret to the fountain of youth* can be found within you. *You* can turn your clock back. Best of all, it's never too late to start. Now is a good time, don't you think?

CHAPTER SIX

IMPROVE YOUR MOOD

Are we in the midst of a depression epidemic? I say yes—and I'd go even further and add anxiety to that. So many of the patients I see, especially women, are struggling to find their happy place in life and struggle to remember what it's like to wake up looking forward to something. Here are the numbers: Almost one out of ten American adults have depression at any given time. Of those, 8.4% have major (clinical) depression, the most serious form. And the rates of depression among women are significantly higher. In fact, women are twice as likely to suffer from depression than men.[1]

It's no surprise, then, that antidepressants are the most prescribed drugs for adults ages 18 to 44, or that a whopping 13.2% of all Americans over age 18 are on one of these medications. Half a million children and adolescents receive prescriptions for them every year.

What is surprising is how well these drugs work—or rather, how well they *don't work*. Despite their enormous popularity, antidepressants aren't all that helpful. Less than half of people who take an antidepressant see their depression disappear, and many stop taking the drugs due to side effects such as weight gain and loss of libido.[2]

Life with depression is both unhappy and physically damaging. It unleashes a cascade of biological and behavioral effects that can worsen just about every aspect of your health. Fortunately, the answer to "Do I have to feel like this forever?" is an emphatic "NO."

Depression always loomed in Thalia's life. At 60 years old, she could not remember a time when she was happy. By her recollection, she had felt "weighed down" and sad since childhood. Thalia grew up an only child with an emotionally absent mother who suffered from bipolar disorder. Her mother's moods were unpredictable and Thalia never felt safe. As she grew older, her depression worsened. Medications, including antidepressants, didn't help. She was hospitalized multiple times and was treated with electroshock therapy, and still, Thalia's depression persisted. She came to see me as a last-ditch effort to find a treatment that would work.

To get to the root of the problem I began with an in-depth physical evaluation. I wanted to know if there was a physiological cause for Thalia's depression, such as hypothyroidism (low thyroid). We also dug into her family history: how she grew up, and her life now. I wanted to get a sense of her emotional landscape and figure out how I might be able to help. Our conversations proved illuminating.

Thalia was hypothyroid and she was not processing folic acid properly, both of which can contribute to depression. Hypothyroidism occurs commonly, especially as we age, which is why it is important for every depressed patient to be evaluated with thyroid function blood tests. Treatment for the thyroid condition can often resolve the mood issue. In addition, when certain vitamin levels such as C, D, B, and folate are low, they also can affect mood, so stabilizing these levels can improve depression. For Thalia, these tests gave us a treatment plan I felt confident would help. First, I normalized her thyroid levels with thyroid medication. A genetic test showed her ability to metabolize folic acid, a B vitamin, was impaired, so I prescribed 15 milligrams of L-methylfolate.

Emotionally, Thalia was grappling with significant past and present trauma. I gave her a prescription for a small amount of Prozac and recommended Eye Movement Desensitization and Reprocessing (EMDR) treatment, an effective trauma therapy treatment I will address later in this chapter. Thalia's EMDR sessions helped her resolve her issues with her mother. By taking care of her medical issues, supplementing her with vitamins and thyroid medications, and having her receive psychotherapy, it was my hope that Thalia would be able to climb out of the deep hole of depression where she had resided most of her life.

About a month later, I received a phone call from Thalia. She told me she was happy for the first time in her life! She told me it was like seeing in technicolor instead of black and white. Thalia felt her new outlook on life was nothing short of a miracle, but I knew it was a combination of good medicine, psychology, and proper supplementation.

Our mood is influenced by several factors, and we can do many things to elevate it and feel great. As we saw with Thalia's story, lifestyle, physiological, and emotional factors are all at play when it comes to your mood. A careful evaluation of those factors is essential. In this chapter, I explain the many ways we can optimize and supplement our nutrition to elevate our mood and avoid depression. For those who have experienced trauma, I explain the process and benefits of EMDR, a relatively quick and highly effective therapy, and I get into some fun ways to deal with mood issues, especially social anxiety.

To start, it is important to understand the intimate relationship between the heart, the gut, and the brain, which is best illustrated by looking at mood and depression. Genetics are at play, yes, but your mood generates from a loop that can start in any of these three organ systems of the body.

For example, heart attack and stroke victims often become depressed after their events, and those with an unbalanced microbiome can develop depression, stroke, and heart disease.[3] If the brain has been damaged, it can cause a drop in the "good mood" hormones such as dopamine, oxytocin, and serotonin, which can affect the heart and the gut through the vagus nerve. If the heart has been damaged, the brain and gut will feel it; the brain won't get the nourishment it needs, and the vagus nerve will communicate with the enteric nervous system in the gut, disrupting hormone balance. And, if there is an imbalance in the microbiome, it can lower serotonin and dopamine levels and cause depression.[4] So, if we want to stop a negative mood cycle, keeping the brain and heart healthy is essential. Balancing the gut is crucial too, since that is where most serotonin is made, a hormone that plays a major role in stabilizing our mood. The interesting thing about the mood and gut is that it isn't just about what you eat. It can be about the vitamins you make in the gut. It could also be about the vitamins you do or do not absorb, as Thalia's story exemplifies beautifully. In order to boost your mood, we'll begin by exploring a powerful but often overlooked therapy that EVERYONE needs to know about: L-methylfolate.

The L-Methylfolate Miracle

Thalia's depression, like many people's, was rooted to some degree in genetics. In her case, she had two mutations on a very important gene. The gene, called methylenetetrahydrofolate reductase, or MTHFR, codes for an essential enzyme. Without it, you won't have enough of the feel-good hormone serotonin.[5]

The enzyme in question turns folic acid, also known as vitamin B9, into L-methylfolate, an active form of the vitamin. L-methylfolate has a lot of essential functions. The one that affects mood is helping the body produce the brain chemicals serotonin, norepinephrine, and dopamine (collectively known as neurotransmitters), which play a critical role in mood regulation.

In short, defects in the MTHFR gene mean too little serotonin— and not enough happiness. It turns out these defects are prevalent. Scientists have reported finding as many as 40 different mutations on MTHFR! And in the United States, up to 60% of us have a mutation in one copy of the gene (remember, you have two copies of every gene, one from each parent). Up to 25% of people have at least one mutation on both copies. Having one mutation reduces your ability to convert folic acid by 34%. Having two mutations reduces it by 71%![6]

The treatment is simple: a regular daily dose of L-methylfolate. Yes, a vitamin—you don't even need a prescription! Taken in the right amounts (7.5 to 15 milligrams per day), it can improve mild depression relatively quickly. In a study of depressed elderly patients, the response rate at six weeks was an astounding 81%. Results are often seen in just two weeks.[7]

Adding L-methylfolate was a big piece of improving Thalia's mood. Who would have guessed that it is one of the keys to making serotonin and other "feel good" hormones? The kicker is that you must be genetically programmed to make it. If not, you must take it as a supplement.

If you're taking an antidepressant and aren't getting enough relief, taking L-methylfolate might help. A 2012 study of people with major depression found adding 15 milligrams of the supplement to an antidepressant regimen doubled the improvement in depression symptoms over a period of 30 days.[7]

L-methylfolate is well tolerated, causing no more side effects than a placebo.[8] And it doesn't interact with other medications. The results I've seen are impressive. When I treat people who have MTHFR mutations—even people who aren't depressed—with L-methylfolate, their mood improves. They may find they feel happier and are better able to handle daily stress and, they often sleep better. Related problems such as irritable bowel syndrome will usually get better as well.

If you are depressed, whether you take an antidepressant or not, ask your doctor to test you for an MTHFR defect. All it takes is a blood sample or cheek swab. If your serotonin levels are genetically low, why not find out if a simple vitamin supplement can boost them? The test is Medicare approved and is no longer considered experimental. Most insurance companies cover the MTHFR blood test, and a few will even cover the cheek swab.

• • •

However...

• • •

When it comes to depression, It would be insulting to think a handful of supplements and drugs is all it takes and—*voila!*—you're cured. Depression and mood disorders are complex and complicated, and treating them effectively requires a more holistic approach. There are many factors to consider.

EMDR: Help for Coping with Past Trauma

Depression is complicated. Genes, lifestyle choices, past experiences, and even diet and exercise can affect our moods. Tackling depression requires more than just physical solutions. I have found psychotherapy can be very helpful for some patients, along with other modalities.

Often, I find people who are depressed suffer from symptoms of post-traumatic stress disorder (PTSD). They have had a trauma that influences how they see the world. Some have been molested and abused, some have witnessed horrible events, and some have experienced things that would boggle anyone's mind. For that reason, I often recommend EMDR therapy.

Gail is a 65-year-old woman who raised her grandson Travis on her own. They were very close and, as a boy, he saved his money and bought her a gold necklace for her birthday. When he turned 18, she bought him a pickup truck as a gift. One night not long after, he rolled the truck, hit a tree, and was killed. Gail was devastated. She came to see me two years after the event, and still could not stop crying. I suggested EMDR therapy. Gail fought me tooth and nail; the cost was too high, she didn't think it would help, and she didn't want to talk about her grief with yet another person. But Gail recognized her pain was unbearable, so she finally went.

It took four sessions. At her final session, Gail's therapist suggested she take off the necklace Travis had given her. Gail's response was an emphatic *"No way!"* She was adamant; that would never happen. After that last session, Gail came to see me and proclaimed the therapy hadn't worked. "Well, you're no longer crying," I pointed out, "that's a start." There were other changes, too. Gail typically came to our appointments dressed in drab, gray clothes; that day, she was dressed in a smart purple blouse. She had brushed her hair. Gail realized, and finally admitted, that she did indeed feel stronger.

Six months later, Gail came for a visit. The necklace was off. She was happy and agreed EMDR was the best thing she had ever done. She was able to remember her grandson with love and focus on her happy memories of him.

EMDR, eye movement desensitization reprocessing, is an established therapy psychologists use to help resolve PTSD. It's based on the theory that strong emotions during a traumatic event can interrupt the normal information processing that happens when a memory is formed. Basically, in the moment of trauma, the sympathetic nervous system becomes overwhelmed. As a result, the memory is never fully processed by the brain, and the extremely unpleasant emotions of the moment, and even the physical sensations, are stored along with the memory. The goal of EMDR is to help the patient fully process the memory so it's stored appropriately in the brain—without the over-the-top or inappropriate emotions and physical responses the memory currently evokes. It is remarkable and effective for people who've experienced major traumas and may also help those who have been through less dramatic but still upsetting experiences.[9]

EMDR is a complex process, but it boils down to this: the patient is asked to summon a mental image of the distressing event. As she focuses on that mental image, she follows with her eyes the therapist's fingers, which move side to side across her field of vision, usually for about 30 seconds. EMDR practitioners explain these eye movements disrupt working (short-term) memory and create a state like lucid dreaming. Eventually, after the process is repeated several times, the patient should feel no distress when conjuring the memory.

At that point, the therapist repeats the eye movement exercises as the patient thinks of a more positive memory or belief. Essentially,

EMDR takes the "fear charge" from memories, says Jan Baker, Ph.D., the clinical psychologist to whom I refer patients. "After releasing the fear charge, the person feels detached from any strong negative emotions associated with that experience," says Baker, who specializes in EMDR. She notes therapies like EMDR can help when talk therapy can't. "The 'shock imprint' of the experience is so deep in the nervous system verbal therapy just won't do it." In her practice, it usually takes three or four sessions to "dissolve" the memory circuit associated with the traumatic event. "It literally changes people's lives."

More than a dozen good-quality studies have shown EMDR to be helpful, and it's been recognized as an effective treatment by organizations such as the American Psychiatric Association and the Department of Defense.[10]

If you want to try this form of therapy, ask your doctor for a referral, call the EMDR institute, or go to their website at www.EMDR.com. Dr. Baker recommends you find someone in your area who has had two levels of certification and many years of experience with the therapy.

We've talked about treatments you can do with a specialist, but what can you do on your own to improve your mood? Read on to discover therapies that work for my patients that can be used alone or in conjunction with antidepressants.

Is Your Diet Making You Depressed?

Depression can be due partly to genetics, but lifestyle choices, including diet, can play a major role. This is where we get into the "real meat" of what is driving it…so to speak! Remember, the documentary Supersize Me? The director and star, Morgan Spurlock, was a fit, happy guy who was feeling great. Then he decided to eat McDonalds three times a day for a month and document the effects. During that month, he noticed significant changes in his body and became moody and depressed. It is best that you hear about his experience from Mr. Spurlock himself (Spoiler alert: It is disturbing):

"Interesting, in only thirty days of eating nothing but McDonald's I gained twenty-four and a half pounds, my liver turned to fat and my cholesterol shot up sixty-five points. My body fat percentage went from eleven to eighteen percent, still below the national average of twenty-two percent for men and thirty percent for women. I nearly doubled my risk of coronary heart disease, making myself twice as likely to have heart failure. I felt depressed and exhausted most of the time, my mood swung on a dime and my sex life was non-existent. I craved this food more and more when I ate it and got massive headaches when I didn't. In my final blood test, many of my body functions showed signs of improvement, but the doctors were less than optimistic."[11]

This account is disturbing for so many reasons. Just imagine what can happen over a lifetime if this is what happened to him in just 30 days. It took so little time for him to go from being a happy healthy guy to a miserable, aching mess of a man teetering on the brink of heart and liver failure.

Much of this can be attributed to the change that occurred in his microbiome. The fast food really messed up the whole system.

What About the Microbiome?

Scientists have found that a healthy gut through the microbiome transmits brain signals via the gut neural network known as the enteric nervous system. It exerts behavioral control both under stable and stressful conditions. In depression, there is a dysregulation of these pathways. This is what happened to Morgan Spurlock's gut which, admittedly, is an anecdotal report. But there is more evidence when looking at research studies of patients with Inflammatory Bowel Disease (IBD). Twenty percent had sleep disturbances and depression. Knowing that inflammation of the gut affects the brain and imbalance can cause negative mood changes, research has focused on finding specific microbes that could be playing a role in this.[12]

Diets lacking the proper nutrients to improve mood can cause the microbiome to become unbalanced. A research paper published in 2022 describes a particular bacterium present in depressed patients and not in those who are healthy. Known as Faecalibacterium prausnitzii, it may be the key to curing or at least reducing the level of depression. Knowing about the presence of this bacterium makes it possible to use it diagnostically and then develop treatments to normalize the gut in depressed patients. Fecal transplant, where the unhealthy microbiome is replaced with a healthy one with the introduction of healthy stool from a donor through a colonoscope, may be another option.[13]

Of course, the microbiome can be altered in a healthy way by changing your diet.

It took Morgan Spurlock eating a vegan diet for 14 months to recover. His case was extreme. In those less extreme cases with dietary indiscretions or antibiotics, it can take up to 6 months for the microbiome to recover.[14] The truth is that you don't have to have supersized yourself to feel the effects of a poor diet, especially if that diet is lacking the following nutrients linked to mood.

The B-Happy Vitamins

One problem with a McDonald's-type diet is a lack of folate. Folate, also known as folic acid or vitamin B9, found in green leafy vegetables, nuts, and fruits, is important to produce brain chemicals such as serotonin, dopamine, and norepinephrine. In one study, a third of depressed adults were found to have low levels of folic acid. Another study showed that when depressed patients on Prozac were given a folic acid supplement, their depression improved significantly more than those who didn't take the supplement.[15]

The solution for most people is simple: Eat more fruits and leafy greens. If you're eating plenty of vegetables, you probably don't need a supplement. If you need one, ask your doctor about taking a B-complex supplement that provides folic acid and other B vitamins. One good product is Super B-Complex by Nature Made.

Of course, if a genetic test shows you have an MTHFR mutation (discussed earlier in this chapter), you'll need supplements of L-methylfolate, the active form of folic acid.

Vitamin B12 is another "B happy" vitamin. A hamburger diet may provide plenty of B12, since red meat is a good source, but too much red meat could eventually kill you. Other better-for-you animal products that contain B12 include chicken, fish, seafood, and eggs. If you take a proton-pump inhibitor such as Prilosec (to reduce stomach acid) or birth control pills, you may be prone to B12 deficiency. In addition, many people start to have trouble absorbing B12 from food as they age.

If a blood test shows your levels are low and you suspect one of your medications is to blame, a B-complex supplement might solve the problem. If you're older, consider taking B12 strips that melt under your tongue, available at health-food stores. With these strips, absorption in the stomach isn't an issue. The other alternative is B12 shots. (A spray is also available, but it's ridiculously expensive.)

The daily recommended intake of B12 for adults is 2.4 micrograms, and it's a good idea to have your proper amount for many reasons. Having adequate B12 levels is important for mood and probably for the treatment of depression as well. A study of 115 people in Finland who were being treated for depression found that people with higher levels of B12 responded better to treatment with an antidepressant over six months than those with lower levels.[16]

One last B vitamin, vitamin B6, or pyridoxine, is also important for the formation of serotonin. If you take birth control pills, your levels of B6 may be low. I tell all my patients on oral contraceptives to take a vitamin B supplement. If you're not on the pill and you are a healthy eater with a diet that includes green leafy vegetables, bananas, nuts and seeds, beans, and fish (such as tuna and salmon), then you probably do not need a supplement. A survey in the United States found teenagers and young adults (between ages 21 and 44) are most likely to be deficient.[17]

The RDA for vitamin B6 is 1.3 milligrams for adults 19 to 50, 1.7 milligrams for men 51 and older, 1.5 milligrams for women 51 and older, 1.9 milligrams for pregnant women, and 2 milligrams for breastfeeding women.[18]

D Is for Depression

A 2017 study found vitamin D helped reverse moderate to severe depression in women with type 2 diabetes who had a D deficiency.[19] Although the study was small, the results were significant. Over 12 weeks, when women's vitamin D levels were increased from a range of 8.9 to 14.5 nanograms per milliliter (ng/ml) to between 32 and 38 ng/ml, their depression test scores markedly improved. A larger study would be welcomed, but there are already enough good reasons to maintain a healthy vitamin D level for general health.[20] It is important for strong bones and overall health.

There is no one-size-fits-all recommendation for vitamin D supplements. Some people are better at making and storing vitamin D than others. Some of us live in places that get more sunlight or spend more time outdoors than our peers. (Incidentally, you can't get vitamin D through glass since UVB rays that carry it do not penetrate glass). And if you cover all your exposed skin with sunscreen, it doesn't matter how sunny it is, you'll have a hard time making vitamin D. But taking too much D is dangerous. Unlike water-soluble vitamins, which are excreted if you take too much, D is stored in the liver. Ask your doctor to test your blood levels of D before supplementing.

C Yourself Happier

Low levels of vitamin C have been associated with depression. When researchers compared the vitamin C levels of depressed women who attempted suicide to those of women who were not depressed, their levels were significantly lower.[21] More evidence: A 2008 study at McGill University found people hospitalized with an acute illness or medical problem who were given vitamin C twice daily showed a 34% improvement in their mood scores. Seventy-four percent of the patients were vitamin C deficient at the outset.[22]

It's not hard to maintain adequate vitamin C levels; just eat plenty of colorful fruits (especially citrus fruits, berries, and melons) and vegetables (especially broccoli, bell peppers, and dark, leafy greens). Notice I said *fruits* and not fruit juice, which is loaded with sugar.

Fish Oil: Not Fishy at All

Depression has been linked to inflammation in the body, both as a cause and a result. Omega-3 fatty acids, found in fatty fish, are highly anti-inflammatory. They're also highly concentrated in the brain and are thought to be essential for healthy brain function. It's little wonder that countries with higher fish consumption have less depression and bipolar disorder (a severe form of depression). Plenty of studies link eating fish or taking fish oil supplements with a lowered risk of depression. For example:

- In northern Finland, a study of more than 5,000 people found that women who ate fish regularly were 2.5 times less likely to become depressed than those who rarely ate fish.[23]

- One study gave patients with bipolar disorder ten grams (a huge amount) of fish oil a day or placebo. The results showed that 64% of the patients improved on fish oil compared to 19 percent of those given a placebo.[24]

- A study in Belgium looking at fish oil levels found levels were low in patients with depression. Giving patients fish oil helped to improve their mood.[25]

Fish oil improves blood flow to the brain. It also decreases the amount of arachidonic acid, a type of unhealthy fatty acid, in the brain. Arachidonic acid is a marker for silent inflammation, and there's more of it in the cerebrospinal fluid (the fluid that bathes the brain) of depressed patients.

So how can you get enough fish oil? My first choice is always getting nutrients from food. Aim for two 3-ounce servings of fatty cold-water fish a week, such as salmon, halibut, or herring. Large fish such as tilefish, mackerel, shark, and swordfish contain higher levels of mercury and toxins and need to be eaten in moderation. Catfish and tilapia contain higher levels of unhealthy fatty acids. Farm raised fish may contain pesticides and antibiotics, so I recommend wild fish.

Most of us have a hard time finding fresh wild fish year-round, so it becomes difficult to eat fish twice weekly. In addition, eating ten grams of fish oil daily to treat bipolar disorder can be downright impossible. Fortunately, most fish oil supplements in the United States are mercury-free. They will say it on the label. Good-quality fish oil will contain adequate amounts of docosahexaenoic acid, or DHA (at least 600 milligrams), and eicosatetraenoic acid, or EPA (at least 400 milligrams). These are the fatty acids that are good for you. When you buy fish oil, look at the back label and add the DHA and EPA amounts; the total will tell you how much beneficial fatty acid you're getting.

I've found the Nordic Natural and Eskimo Oil brands of fish oil are best. I recommend at least 1,000 milligrams daily, possibly more based on your mood issues. Check with your doctor before taking fish oil supplements since they can interact with some medications and thin the blood.

Other Therapeutic Supplements

There are so many supplements advertised and on shelves at health food stores and there are plenty of sales personnel ready to tell you how great they are. But are they? Probably not. Minerals and vitamins are essential for our health and are best obtained the truly natural way…through food, not from a pill. Supplements are not regulated the way medications are. They may not contain what they say they do and some can interact with medications. They may have contaminants and the product may not even be available to your body; because many supplements are not absorbed, they end up unchanged in septic tanks and sewers.

According to Grand View Research, they do bring in a lot of money though; 151.9 billion dollars reportedly in 2021. Very expensive waste, don't you think?[26]

Keeping this in mind, there are several over-the-counter supplements touted to help with depression—I recommend only two, and my recommendation is measured. Because, while they can be effective, it's important to know about these popular supplements before you try them.

St. John's Wort has been shown in most studies to help with mild to moderate depression. A potential downside of taking this herb is it interacts with many medications. For this reason, it is important to avoid taking it with antidepressants. Another significant problem is the amount of the most important ingredient, hypericin, can vary widely from one brand to the next, so it's very hard to know when or if you're getting a therapeutic dose.[27]

The second supplement, SAMe, is popular for depression, and some studies show it does work. There's also evidence it can boost the effectiveness of antidepressants. I prescribe it for joint health more than mental health. I don't recommend it often because it gets awfully expensive—well over $100 a month—if you take the dosages that help with depression.

By now you have gotten the idea that I am leery of supplements and often medications when it comes to treating depression.[28] I am always in search of ways for patients to find the healthiest pathways out of a depression that will serve them well in the long run. Sometimes the use of medication is unavoidable but there is often another way. Exercise is one of those healthy paths.

Exercise as an Antidepressant

Regular exercise makes us feel good physically. It can also help with depression. In a landmark study done in 1999, researchers took 156 men and women and divided them into three groups.

One group followed an aerobic exercise program, another took the antidepressant Zoloft, and a third did both. At the end of 16 weeks, they all had improved. In fact, 60 to 70%of people across all the groups were no longer considered to have major depression. This means the exercise worked as well as the antidepressant (with fewer side effects)! After six months, the researchers checked in with the patients again and found those in the exercise-only group were less likely to have relapsed than those who took medication and didn't exercise.[29]

What kind of exercise is for you? The kind you're most likely to keep doing! Find something you like and make it part of your life. It could be bicycling, running, hiking, or dancing. The key is to get moving and keep moving. The more you exercise, the better you'll feel.

Improve Your Mood The Fun Way!

It's no secret exercise is good for you, but it does relieve depression. Studies have repeatedly proven this for decades to the point that it's almost common knowledge.

Better than Zoloft? Yes!

In *Understanding Depression*, a 2011 Harvard Medical School Special Health Report, doctors explain the benefits of exercise on depression and cite a 1999 study that shows regular exercise is at least as effective as antidepressants, such as Zoloft. For patients with depression who need or wish to avoid drugs, exercise might be an acceptable substitute for antidepressants. Even better, a follow-up to that study found the positive effects of exercise lasted longer than those of antidepressants.[30]

In a similar study, researchers found 30 minutes of brisk exercise three times a week is just as effective as drug therapy in relieving the symptoms of major depression in the short term. Continued exercise greatly reduces the chances of depression returning.[31]

Another study published in 2014 directly explained this phenomenon of happiness cultivated by dancing. Researchers discovered the Argentine Tango worked as well as if not better than mindfulness meditation for relieving stress and depression. In the study, 66 participants were divided into three groups. One group took Tango classes, the other was assigned to meditate, and the third was placed on a waiting list. Depression levels were reduced for both the Tango and meditation groups. Interestingly, only the Tango group achieved significantly reduced stress levels.[32] One of my patients found that dance was his best medicine for depression. Here is his story:

Joe is 62, extremely fit, and an avid dancer. His favorites are West Coast Swing and Country 2-Step. He is trim and muscular; he looks like he's ready to run a marathon. He is married and very happy. He's been dancing for about two-and-a-half years.

He first started dancing to improve his social life. He found he liked it and it got him out of his shell. In the beginning, it was tough. Everything hurt and he wondered if he was too old to dance. But he liked the music and decided to take a private lesson. He contemplated quitting at various points, but he had found a dance partner, and the two kept each other going.

He has mastered dancing enough now that it has become his regular aerobic workout. It allows him exercise, creativity, and fun. Most importantly, it is good for his mental and physical health. Joe describes himself as a recovering alcoholic; he has not had a drink in 25 years. Prone to depression, dance has been a godsend.

Not only does the movement contribute to his elevated mood, the fun he has doing it is also a huge help. He used to be very self-conscious about dancing, but now he is much better both with his dancing and his confidence. He knows dance provides the gift of health and wellbeing. He often dances at a place where he has seen people in their 80s, 90s, and even 100s dancing and that provides him with continued motivation and inspiration.

How Exactly Does Exercise Work
To Overcome Depression?

The answer is endorphins. These chemicals have been naturally occurring within us for millennia but have only started to be understood since the 1970s. Scientists discovered the human body makes its own version of morphine and named these chemicals accordingly: "endorphin" was coined by combining the words endogenous, meaning "proceeding from within; derived internally," and the pain-killer morphine. The researchers combined the endo from endogenous and the orphin from morphine to describe these newly discovered chemicals, endorphins, the body's self-made feel-good drugs.[33]

Endorphins pretty much work as advertised by their names. They are analgesics our bodies produce naturally. They kick in when we exercise intensely for an "endorphin rush" or a "runner's high." However, they are elevated and then stick around for higher and sustained feelings of happiness and well-being with regular, moderate exercise. Again, studies show that's just about 30 minutes a day a few times a week. So, how come everybody isn't exercising regularly and feeling great?

As you know, it's tough to stick to exercising. It is statistically likely that you have started and then abandoned a workout plan. Over 50% of people who join a gym quit within the first 6 months.[34] Post pandemic, 56% of people are working out online.[35] That leaves hundreds of thousands of people who enthusiastically begin well-thought-out programs of diets and exercise, only to drop them a few weeks or a couple of months later. Why is that?

Why do people keep failing with their diets and exercise? It's pretty simple, really. It's hard to keep going, and it's not much fun. Ever look around the gym at the faces in the weight room or the aerobics studio? How about the face of a runner? It's tough to find anyone smiling or looking the least bit pleased in these situations.

That's because they're not particularly happy "in the moment." Most people who are working out are in it for the secondary effect.

In other words, they take their medicine because they know it's good for them, but they're not enjoying the taste of that medicine; they do it only for the cumulative benefit of good health and well-being they know it provides.

Unfortunately for many, this delayed gratification benefit of good health is simply not enough to overcome the unpleasantness, hassle, and pain of regular exercise. Hence, the very high dropout rate.

Dancing Is The Answer!

Dancing is fun, social, relatively inexpensive, and has a very low injury rate, it's much easier for many people to stick with it. And it's a great workout. The World DanceSport Federation (WDSF) refers to lead and follow dancing as a sport and its dancers as athletes. The International Olympic Committee agrees, having granted Ballroom dancing full recognition as a sport in 1997.[36]

Dance is a great low-impact exercise that gives a total body workout. It is mentally as well as physically demanding, and it is exciting and engaging. When Dr. Jill McNitt-Gray, professor of kinesiology and biological sciences at the University of Southern California, was asked by ABC's Dancing with the Stars to come on the show and explain some of the findings of recent scientific research regarding the level of fitness of dancers. She confirmed that: "Dancers are some of the toughest athletes in the world."[36]

The good news is you don't have to be a professional dancer to get the benefits from dancing. Among the many gains one can enjoy from dancing, the mental health component may be the greatest.

What If You Need Medication?

Even after eating a clean diet and exercising, some people may still need medication. If that is the case, it is often hard to determine which drug to choose. I had always wondered how nice it would be if there was a road map or manual. Now, I have found the solution. There is a genetic test that gives me a framework of medications to work with. It helps me see which medications a patient metabolizes normally and which they do not. This test extends to antipsychotics, anxiolytics, and medicine for ADD and ADHD. I will explain.

We are all born with a unique makeup of genes that code our DNA. As I explained earlier, they code for everything; our sex, our appearance, and how our body works. Genes also code for the enzymes that break down drugs in our liver. Many medications are metabolized there. An entire system of enzymes called Cytochrome P450 does the work. The gene test I do with a simple cheek swab, called GeneSight, determines the unique way the major enzymes of the liver metabolize the drugs that go through this system. It looks at the individual enzyme activity and multiple enzymes' activity that may impact how we metabolize a particular drug.[37]

This test has been literally a lifesaver for many. There is no way to look at someone and tell if a drug will be harmful to them. By looking at how things are metabolized, I have a much better idea. The test will tell me if someone is a normal, slow, rapid, or ultra-rapid metabolizer. If they are normal, there is a lower risk of an adverse reaction. If they are a slow metabolizer, they may experience side effects at the usual dose of a medication, and it may not work very well. If they are a rapid or an ultra-rapid metabolizer, the drug may not build up a blood level of the medication so it can work at the usual dosage; thus, more may be needed.

With a very simple printout, I can see if a drug has a high likelihood of causing a significant reaction. If so, it would be in the red zone. If it is questionable, it is in the yellow zone, and if it doesn't have a known gene-drug interaction, it is in the green zone.

In full disclosure, I have been so impressed with the test results that I speak for the company to educate other physicians about it. I have been paid an honorarium, but I would do it regardless because this test has revolutionized my practice.

It is incredible how many people were getting sick from the medications that were supposed to help them to get better. I had one patient on so many medications she wasn't metabolizing that she felt normal again when I stopped them all. That is what was making her sick. I now do the test before I start a patient on any antidepressant.

I highly recommend this test if you are on antidepressants or contemplating going on them. If you have children who need medication for depression or ADD/ADHD, this test is essential. Ritalin is the usual medication, but studies have found 30% of those started on it will have an adverse reaction.[38] The test is easy to do. Think about it. The test is useful in finding the proper treatment for depression and for anxiety, a growing problem since the COVID-19 pandemic.

Anxiety

Anxiety is a stress reaction. The best way to look at it is that stress is external, and anxiety is internal. It triggers the outpouring of the "Fight or Flight" stress hormones, and we feel it. At one point or another, all of us have experienced anxiety. It is normal and keeps us safe but, if it is continuous, we develop chronic anxiety. Unfortunately, the pandemic has caused many more to experience continuous stress and develop chronic anxiety. In fact, 4 in 10 adults in the US reported having anxiety or depressive disorders during the pandemic versus 1 in 10 who reported it prior to the pandemic. They have experienced difficulty with sleep (36%), eating (32%) and reported an increase in substance abuse (12%). That is why it is so important that we learn how to deal with our stress in constructive ways. Once again, healthy eating and a balanced microbiome are the answer.[39]

A review of 21 articles published in 2019 showed an overall positive effect on anxiety symptoms by regulating the gut microbiota. Fifty-two percent of the studies showed that this was effective. Five used probiotic supplements and six used non-probiotic interventions. Six of seven studies showed an 86% reduction of anxiety.[40]

Another form of anxiety that has been present and worsened since the pandemic is known as social anxiety. This disorder is characterized by fear and anxiety that lead to avoidance of social situations. It can affect every aspect of life. As people return to the "new normal" post-pandemic, this type of anxiety has been magnified. Now that we can get together with people, there is a non-threatening, non-medication-based solution.

Dance Social Anxiety Away!

Consider the last wedding reception you attended. When it was time for the guests to dance, you likely saw only a few venture out onto the floor (the brave, the crazies, and the drunks). After a while, some others were coaxed and cajoled and eventually got their courage up and reluctantly started to dance, while others refused to be dragged out under any circumstances—or they simply hid in the corner or up and left when the dancing started. As rocker Morrissey of The Smiths wrote, "Shyness can stop you from doing all the things in life you'd like to." Social anxiety can be utterly debilitating.

No matter where one may be placed on the spectrum, from a case of shyness to true social anxiety (SA), the mere idea of dancing strikes fear into the hearts (and feet) of many. What's this about? Why are some people so averse to dancing? Insecurity. No one wants to feel awkward or stupid or be laughed at. Some people go their whole lives avoiding dancing; if they must dance, it's only when forced and/or inebriated. For others, the social anxiety they feel daily not only puts dancing completely out of the question but also makes most social situations stressful. Parties, groups of people, public gatherings, or celebrations are not things to be enjoyed but endured or (preferably) avoided entirely. I have a friend who has experienced it for most of her life and found a way to overcome it. Here is her story.

Uchiki was a very shy, reserved girl by nature. In addition, she was raised with a traditional Japanese ethos, which meant any kind of extroversion was frowned upon. As a grown woman in America, she was still always the quiet one. Although she couldn't admit it to herself at the time, she lived her life walled off from being how she truly wanted to be, from being her true self. For Uchiki, dancing changed everything.

One day, a friend saw Uchiki moving to a song at a party and asked her to come to a dance lesson with her. After weeks of relentless prodding, Uchiki reluctantly went. She was surprised to find she really liked it. And she realized an added benefit: she could be social without talking to anyone.

The toughest part of dancing for Uchiki was touching a man's hand and making eye contact. The more she danced, the easier it was to overcome that hurdle. She realizes dancing has made her feel free to be who she truly is. Her life had consisted of caring for her grandmother, mother, husband, and son. However, her marriage ended (amicably) and her son grew up and left home. She found herself with new and unfamiliar freedom and the opportunity arose to enjoy it. Dancing has given her a new life. It has opened an entirely new group of friends and dance partners. Uchiki has come out of her shell, can make eye contact, and occasionally flirt. For Uchiki, dance is love, joy, and gratitude.

You don't have to be diagnosed with a full-blown case of social anxiety to benefit from its strategies and treatments. According to the experts, shyness and SA are part of the same continuum. Social anxiety is simply more severe. Even if you just struggle occasionally with shyness or self-esteem, you can be helped.

With the above in mind, evidence confirms that SA is successfully treated through dance. Dr. Thomas A. Richards, Ph.D., psychologist, and founder of the Social Anxiety Institute, talks about the importance of using Cognitive–Behavioral Therapy (CBT) to treat SA. CBT teaches people how to reformat their thoughts in a positive light. A big part of the therapy is being proactive; taking the initiative rather than just reacting when things happen to you in life. Group dance lessons can give people an opportunity to do that. The student can relax and focus on learning. It is a safe and comfortable environment. Everyone is in the same boat.[41]

One of the experts on social anxiety, Dr. Bill Knaus, created an interesting workshop that included an exercise called the "Shy Away." Participants were asked to pantomime shyness through their dancing and gestures. Within seconds on the dance floor, they were all doing the Shy Away. At the end of the exercise, Dr. Knaus asked if anyone would do a dance solo. Not surprisingly, no one volunteered.

What did each learn from the experience? Dr. Knaus heard many perspectives. Some were amazed they could do it. Many realized how much fun they had when they loosened up and danced. Even the most anxious said it wasn't too bad. A few said the exercise was too easy. Most felt neither judged nor threatened. The Shy Away was a breakthrough exercise.

This presents a perfect icebreaker for safe mingling. Having a basic conversation about the shared joys of dance can help anyone with their communication skills and, eventually, their overall social competence.[42]

It may seem counter-intuitive, but the scariest of all possible social situations—dancing in public—is the key to feeling more confident and less awkward in dance and all social situations.

Dancing helps with shyness and social anxiety, that is, how we feel about our interaction with the outside world. Dancing also helps with how we feel about our internal world: our self-confidence. For this, we have to convince ourselves that we can just go ahead and do it.

• • •

Fake it till you make it!

• • •

For many there is a catch–22 regarding a lack of confidence and dancing: sure, dancing builds confidence, but if one needs the confidence to get started dancing to *build* confidence, how can that possibly work? We would all agree that self-confidence is an important ingredient for success. If you don't have it, it is possible to pretend you do have it. Putting on a confident face will allow a person to get through a variety of stress-inducing situations. I know it has helped me! In other words, fake it till you make it! The situations become less scary over time and you will need to fake it less and less.

Of course, there are instances of the extreme; forcing oneself through a very difficult situation, despite the anxiety: the famous dance scene from the movie "Napoleon Dynamite" comes to mind. To help his friend, Pedro, who is running for class president of their high school, Napoleon takes center stage at the school-wide assembly and does an unrehearsed, unchoreographed dance in front of an auditorium full of his disaffected classmates. This audience at first starts out quite unreceptive, sitting stone-silent and staring at him.

We can all relate to this feeling Napoleon must have endured. We all sometimes feel intense pressure and are nervous when facing certain situations. Jon Heder, the actor who plays Napoleon, describes the climactic moment of the film: "Everything leads up to this...this has been the moment where he lands a victory." Napoleon bets it all—and wins. He is cheered and then even receives a standing ovation (and Pedro gets elected).[43]

This phenomenon has been the fodder for many writers. In an interview with Insider Magazine, regarding the iconic dance scene, Jon Heder stated, "Really the Napoleon dance is just dancing from your heart. It's just like, feeling it and just letting it go." Be yourself. It is empowering. The message is: if we face our fears, we too can conquer them and build our self-esteem.[44]

Thankfully, when it comes to dancing, you don't necessarily have to go the route of the all-or- nothing gamble like Napoleon. You have the more comfortable option to take things slowly. You can take lessons with others who likely share some of the same hesitations and concerns and are at a similar skill level. When social dancers achieve a certain level of success, their self-esteem and confidence often improve.

• • •

Floor time is your friend.

• • •

So, there is a flip side to the catch–22. That is, dance builds your confidence, and confidence builds your dance. The smart way to approach it: *floor time is your friend.* Simply stated, the more you dance, the better you get and the better you feel, on and off the floor. It will do great things for your body image and your fitness level, both of which will help to enhance your sex life! In fact, certain dances have been coined as the vertical expression of a horizontal position. This holds true, particularly for tango. Not only does it help get you in the mood, it also helps with communication between couples, if that is a "stumbling block" for you regarding sex.

CHAPTER SEVEN

SEX WILL KEEP YOU HEALTHY

Sex is mostly whispered about behind closed doors. Instead, we should be shouting about it out in the open. It is normal and important for intimate partner relationships, and absolutely nothing to be ashamed of. Whether alone or with a partner, sex is essential for our health and well-being, especially when we look at our buddies, the brain, the heart, and the gut.

LET'S START WITH THE BRAIN

Good sex can make us feel great! With every orgasm, your body releases beneficial chemicals, one of which is a hormone called DHEA. DHEA boosts cognition, strengthens the immune system, and even improves the look of your skin. DHEA also has been found to improve body composition and metabolism in older adults.[1]

Sex releases endorphins, key neurochemicals that help prevent or relieve depression, ease stress and anxiety, improve self-image and help regulate appetite. When our cuddle and bonding hormone oxytocin is released, it acts as a chemical messenger in sexual arousal, trust, and romantic attachment. It also triggers the same feelings of love that occur when moms look into their baby's eyes. It enhances empathy and trust and is vital for bonding in romantic relationships. It does this by producing an after-glow effect that lasts 48 hours. In the first stages of a romance, those levels can stay elevated for up to six months.[2] This is quite a powerful combination, and research suggests that sex and intimacy in a loving relationship are good for the heart.

What About The Heart?

Being healthy and fit are important for a good sexual relationship. Sexual activity is a form of exercise. For some, it is more athletic than for others. I once found a book my son had hidden in his room called *365 Sex Positions: A New Way Every Day*[3]— now that is a book of injuries ready to happen! Many of us would end up in urgent care trying to get into the positions outlined in that book! In fact, that is exactly what happened to a friend of mine. It was hard for her to explain her injury to the young attending doctor, who I am sure was quietly giggling to himself.

But regardless, even standard positions require a bit of flexibility, and the activity promotes all sorts of benefits like cardiovascular health and muscle building. Sex with a known partner is considered mild to moderate activity, the equivalent of climbing two flights of stairs or walking quickly. And like any other form of exercise, sex offers many physical health benefits. A study by the National Institutes of Health found that a half-hour of sexual activity can burn 125 calories for men and 100 calories for women. This is similar to walking at a three-mile-per-hour pace.[4]

A study published in 2010 concurs that sex is good for the heart. Researchers found that men who have an orgasm once a month or less were 45 percent more likely to have a stroke or develop heart disease than those who had sex more than twice weekly. The researchers postulated that men with better overall health had a stronger sex drive which caused them to have more sex and boosted their cardiovascular health.[5]

However, like any form of physical exercise, there are associated risks. In a recent study, women who were in a sexually fulfilling relationship had a lower risk of hypertension five years later. Men had a higher chance of cardiovascular events five years later.[6] And one study found women were unaffected by sexual frequency regarding cardiac status. However, sexually active older men who had sex once a week were more likely to experience coronary events than those who did not.[7] The reason is that they often have trouble achieving orgasm which can cause cardiovascular stress. Medications such as Viagra can also have a negative impact.

A Potential Downside

Another situation that can put men at risk of sudden cardiac death during sexual activity is men who are cheating on their partners. When I was a resident in training, I saw it several times. As the treating physician, it made a tactful discussion difficult. It was hard to explain to the family what happened, especially when the patient was present and he was not forthcoming about the circumstances.

When men meet women, particularly younger women, to have an affair outside their homes, they are at greater risk of suffering a life-threatening cardiac event. However, why this happens is not entirely clear. It could be the adrenaline rush, the stress, or the guilt, but it does happen. That increased risk in men of cardiac arrest during sex could also have something to do with the need for supplements and medications to help with sexual function—increasingly popular in recent decades. Still, they aren't without their side effects. For men who take nitroglycerin, if any of the sex aids such as Cialis or Viagra are used, it can be deadly.[8]

The importance of the heart during sex is understandable. You need a healthy heart to be active in general. Sex as an activity requires the heart "pump" normally. But, what about the gut, and why is it important for sexual activity? It may not be as obvious, but you will see it is very important.

What's The Gut Got To Do With It?

The gut is important for sexual activity because, as we mentioned earlier, 90% of the serotonin in the body is made in the gut. When this level is low, so is your sex drive. Estrogen is also regulated in the gut by the microbiome. The estrogens moderate the vaginal microbiome. That is how they affect each other with conditions such as PCOS and endometriosis.

In addition to having your hormones to deal with in the gut, experiencing discomfort from any number of conditions is a total buzz kill. Who can think about sex if they are constipated or have diarrhea? That is why you want a healthy gut. If it works smoothly, you have a better shot at a good sex life.[9]

As we age, it is more likely that systems can go wrong. The question is, should that interfere with us enjoying healthy sexual relationships? I say, NO.[10]

Age Should Not Be a Limiting Factor

We can see that sex is vital for many things. It is important for overall health and keeps people motivated to pursue a healthy lifestyle. Those with active sex lives are more likely to get regular checkups, take their medication, and adopt healthy habits. They also have more confidence. As to relationships, those with a healthy sex life tend to have a better bond.

Unfortunately, some people feel that sex has an expiration date. It doesn't and, in fact, can get better as we age. A study by the University of Michigan found that 40% of people aged 65-80 are sexually active. Three-quarters of the people studied had a romantic partner. Fifty-four percent were sexually active. Regardless, two-thirds of the entire group surveyed were interested in sex.[11]

One of the obstacles to having sex is a lack of libido. For men, Viagra and Cialis have revolutionized their sex lives. For women, these drugs have been tried, but the side effects just aren't worth it to the women who have tested them.

Is There Something Better to Help Our Libido?

We know from studies that sex makes us healthier and happier. For most, the magic number is once a week for optimal health. More than that can put pressure on a couple and probably does not infer any more physical benefit. In addition to feeling good, you can live longer, too. Here's some important information to help you have better sex and thus enjoy a longer, better life.[12]

Antidepressants put a damper on sexual response and the libido. A study of women taking antidepressants found Viagra improved women's experience by 72% as opposed to 27% by placebo.[13] Unfortunately, women experienced similar side effects as men, including headache, nasal congestion, flushing, nausea, and visual symptoms.[13] While it is clear Viagra can help some women, the side effects may be enough to keep women from trying it.

Fortunately, thanks to my friends, the compounding pharmacists, there is another option: "Scream Cream." It is a mix of Viagra, Aminophylline, and L-Arginine. Some pharmacists may switch out the Aminophylline with nitroglycerin 0.2%. These are compounds that dilate blood vessels and are applied to the clitoral area an hour before sexual activity. It helps improve sensitivity and sexual function, and has helped most of my patients. There are no side effects and we have noted no long-term adverse effects. One of my patients, Sylvia, benefited from this.

Sylvia is a 65-year-old woman who suffered a stroke 3 years ago and was left with some weakness on her left side. Although she regained some strength, she developed a mild depression commonly seen in stroke survivors, which improved with the antidepressant Celexa. She and her husband had always enjoyed a healthy sex life; however, the antidepressant dulled her sensation, and it was hard for her to achieve orgasm. She also noted that increasing vaginal dryness was causing her discomfort.

To improve her sensation, I prescribed Viagra cream, available at our compounding pharmacy as a prescription for the last few years. For the vaginal dryness, I suggested she use vaginal estriol mini-inserts every other night. She applied the cream to her clitoral area about 45 minutes before engaging in intercourse. Her vaginal dryness improved, and her sensation returned. In fact, things went so well that she and her husband enjoyed a "second honeymoon" in Hawaii.

They were having so much fun in bed one night that her screams of ecstasy were mistaken for a brutal attack and, the next thing they knew, the concerned hotel security banged on their door, fearing she was being harmed. They were both quite embarrassed but explained they were just having fun—and coined the term "Scream Cream" for her Viagra!

• • •

Screaming For The Right Reason

• • •

Scream Cream can spice up your sex life. However, if you suffer from vaginal dryness, you may not find it much fun. Twenty to forty percent of women in midlife and beyond suffer from this condition (also known as "vaginal atrophy" in the medical world, but we prefer "dryness" to this rather unkind medical designation).[14] Due to a lack of hormones after menopause, the tissues of the vagina become dry and sex is often painful. There are many treatments and I share here what I have found to be most successful for my patients.

If your doctor determines it is safe for you to use hormones, vaginal estriol is an effective treatment. It is a very weak and relatively safe form of estrogen.[15] It is often used in women who have been treated for breast cancer. I prescribe it as a mini vaginal insert made by a compounding pharmacy in a low dose (0.5 mg) that women use every other night. If your testosterone level is low, it can be added as well. This can improve your libido, and you will find yourself having more fun than you have had in ages!

For a non-hormone solution, I recommend vitamin E vaginal suppositories made by Carlson. Many studies show they work and have no side effects. Carlson also makes fish oil capsules. Don't get them mixed up, like one of my friends did! She inserted the fish oil by mistake. She was in horror at the time, but, needless to say, we later got a good laugh out of that one!

Finally, something else I recommend for dryness is called V-Magic, used on the vulvar area, which we know can become dry as we age. It consists of olive oil, avocado oil, beeswax, sea buckthorn, and organic honey.[16] The combination is healing and soothing. Although it is designed for the vulvar area, many of my patients have used it with great success for cuts, chapped lips, and an abundance of irritated areas.

And For Women Who Have Discomfort For Another Reason

Viagra is a potent vasodilator and has been explored for use in menstrual cramps, which seems to work. A study by Penn State College recruited 25 women to vaginally administer 100 mg of Viagra.[17] They rated their pain over four hours. Those given Viagra were twice as likely to note relief as those given a placebo. There were no side effects reported in either group. Since Viagra vaginal suppositories are unavailable commercially, I have prescribed the compounded version. It has worked exceptionally well and has not caused any adverse effects. If you are a woman incapacitated by your periods due to pain, there is no longer a need to suffer.

As I stated earlier, the above prescriptions require a compounding pharmacy. Discuss them with your doctor. I use the local Wellness Compounding Pharmacy, www.wellnessformyhealth. com. You may also find favorite compounding pharmacy by going to **www.findacompounder.com**.

The Impact Of How We Feel On The Enjoyment Factor

So far, we have addressed the physicality of enjoying sex. We, as women, know that much of our enjoyment involves how we feel about our partner; we need to feel comfortable and cared for. In other words, our most powerful sex organ is our brain. Here is a story:

Fay is a 40-year-old woman who grew up in a family of all women, the eldest of four sisters. Her father left when she was a baby and, as she grew up, she was often left to care for her siblings when her mother worked. Fay had a very limited social life as a teenager and young adult. She went to an all-girls high school. To be close to home, Fay attended a local college where she met and married her first boyfriend. She was head-over-heels for him. They married within six months and Fay moved from her mother's house to his. Initially, things went well. The newlyweds had fun getting to know each other. Sex was new, and she enjoyed herself. Over time, they settled into a routine, both working full-time. Fay did what she was used to and took responsibility for the lion's share of the family chores. She became overwhelmed and started to resent her husband and became withdrawn from him. She was exhausted at night and sex, which had been fun and exciting, no longer appealed to Fay.

Fay came to see me as a patient. After some frank questioning, it turned out she had not discussed her feelings with her husband. He was a very caring man who loved her and was unaware of how burdened she felt. Growing up with women, Fay had little experience speaking to men. I suggested she give it a try, and little by little, she opened up to him and began to ask for help around the house and for time away together. He happily complied, and within about six months, Fay's life had improved, and they were enjoying each other both in and out of the bedroom.

Fay's experience is not unique. I don't need to state the obvious, but I will. Men and women are very different, and we look at things differently. Sometimes (okay, a lot of the time) men baffle us. We are often afraid to approach them about what is bothering us. But it is important.

• • •

Let's Talk!

• • •

Like most things, having a healthy sex life takes work. Here are some tips to guide you.

- First things first: make sure you feel good enough for sex. Address issues that may be causing you to hesitate; joint pain, belly pain, and body aches can all interfere. See your doctor and find out what you can do to feel better.

- As with Fay, discuss relationship issues frankly and honestly. Most women cannot enjoy sex when they are pissed off. For men, it does not seem to be much of an issue. Most are always ready regardless.

- Know what you like by exploring your own body. Find the spots that stimulate you and show your partner. That will be a turn-on in and of itself.

- If things are not going well, don't fake it. That doesn't help either of you. The truth is, men take 4 minutes to reach orgasm. Women take around 10 to 11 minutes. When surveyed 75% of men say they always reach orgasm. Twenty-six percent of women do. When their male partners were asked, they predicted that their female partners achieved orgasm far more often than they actually did.[18] So, the bottom line is, they have no idea. The only way they will know is if you speak up.

- Foreplay is important. Sometimes, just cuddling, laughing and talking are enough to get things started. Cuddling afterward is also important for the relationship. Take full advantage of all that oxytocin you produced!

- Get your timing together. In our busy lives, scheduling sex makes sense, and it can lead to fun anticipation.

- There are always fun things to assist you. People giggle when you talk about sex toys, but they are readily available online and can help. Check out Amazon. There are tons! They are delivered in discreet packages. No reason not to try them. Go with whatever piques your curiosity.

- Masturbation is another option, with or without a partner. Contrary to the nuns from grade school who talked about the evils of masturbation, your hands and other parts won't fall off. It is good for you. It keeps everything in working order and can work as a turn-on for your partner.

Sexual desire and experience differ between men and women. Studies have shown that men tend to have a stronger sex drive and think about it more than women. Most men under 60 tend to think about sex at least once a day, if not more. Only a quarter of women report thinking about sex that often.[19]

What Will It Take?

Men seek out sex more often than women, both at the beginning and throughout the life of a relationship. It does not take much to get most of them turned on. They tend to be more visual. When it comes to women, the key is feeling safe, loved, and comfortable. A boob grab doesn't really do it as a turn-on. We need more of an emotional connection. It seems like having a satisfying sexual relationship ought to be easy, but it is complicated. If you follow the "tips" and things still aren't working for you, therapists are available to help you and your partner.

Sex is important for many things; for overall health and keeping people motivated to pursue a healthy lifestyle. As I said earlier, those with active sex lives are more likely to get regular checkups, take their medication, and adopt healthy habits. They also have more confidence. In terms of relationships, those with a healthy sex life tend to have a better bond. But a word of caution if you are thinking about having sex with a new partner.

STIs

If you are considering a sexual relationship with someone new, remember that sexually transmitted illnesses are out there. You and your potential partner need to be tested, and it is imperative that you talk about your past histories. This is very important since more seniors are having sex. As a result, the incidence of sexually transmitted infections (STIs) is rising. A survey by the CDC found that the highest rises in those over 55 were in Washington DC, New York, and Maryland. These diseases included Chlamydia, gonorrhea, syphilis, and HIV. Please beware![20]

I know the discussion around STIs isn't easy, especially for those over 65, not just with partners but with the medical profession as well. A variety of things can complicate these discussions; embarrassment, negative attitudes, and disinterest by the health professionals can all contribute. Communication is once again key. Be your own advocate AND Please, please, please…USE CONDOMS!

• • •

Communication and the use of condoms are the keys! [21]

• • •

IN CONCLUSION

Sex often becomes a sidebar in our lives, especially as we age. However, you can see how important it is for health. As with anything worthwhile in life, including our brain, heart, and gut health, it takes work. Great sex requires communication and interaction. The benefit is that it enhances relationships, feels good, and is FUN! It is important for life balance as well…

CHAPTER EIGHT

FINDING THE RIGHT BALANCE LITERALLY AND METAPHORICALLY

As we age, balance and the chance of falling can be the difference between life and death. Just one significant fall can be devastating. The statistics are daunting. According to the Centers for Disease Control, three million older people are treated each year in emergency departments for fall injuries and those injuries often have life-changing consequences. Falls are the number one cause of fractures, hospital admissions for trauma, loss of independence, and deaths due to injury. Furthermore, falling once doubles your chances of falling again; a serious fall is rarely just a one–time event.[1]

Why are serious falls such a common phenomenon, especially for older adults? There are several risk factors involved, ranging from poor reactions to certain medications to bone frailty due to a lack of vitamin D. However, two of the biggest contributing factors are a lack of muscle strength and a decline in balance. These two issues are compounded as we age. Many studies show these conditions along with a decline in motor skills, and our ability to react to stimuli, as the reasons for the risks of falling.[2]

The rate at which this happens is variable and does not have to be inevitable. Many older people just give up and decide they don't need to exercise anymore when, in reality, exercise can make all the difference.

Other older individuals lose a little of any skill as they age. But again, it takes work. You can see this with professional musicians such as the Rolling Stones and Itzhak Perlman, and in athletes from diverse sports such as golf and bowling—even powerlifters (male and female, I might add) who continue to lift much heavier-than-average-weight well into their 60s, 70s and even 80s.[3]

What Seems To Make The Difference?
Work, Work, Work!

As they age, musicians learn that they must keep moving and exercise to keep their edge (and to keep those energy levels high on stage). This helps them stay in shape. Flexibility is very important. Many regularly perform endurance activities such as walking, running, and cycling. This helps them maintain their posture, especially those who play instruments in asymmetrical positions, such as the cellist or violinist. They practice consistently and continue to study and work at their craft. Warming up is essential and may take longer than when they were younger. It helps the joints. Being cognizant of technique is also important. They take more breaks and adjust their equipment to fit their needs.[4]

As professional athletes age, many have learned from experience and manage the stress of competition much better than their younger counterparts which tends to counterbalance the physical effects of aging. They may not reverse aging but can significantly slow it down. To do this, cardio is key. The best exercises are endurance types such as running, swimming, bicycling, and high-intensity interval training. Weight training is good for muscle maintenance, but studies keep aerobic exercises at the very top of the list.[5]

Researchers found this when they studied 124 healthy, inactive adults between 30 and 60. They were divided into four groups; one group remained inactive, the other three groups exercised for 45 minutes three times a week for 26 weeks. One group ran or walked, another did high intensity interval training, and the third did resistance training. Interestingly, the endurance (intensity interval) training groups experienced the anti-aging effects of their workout, and the resistance training and inactive groups did not.

The effects were tested by looking at special studies of white blood cells taken before and after the study. Remember the discussion of telomeres on page 103? Telomeres sit at the end of chromosomes and act as protective caps. These types of exercises maintained telomere length in those who exercised and were comparable to people 9 years younger.[6]

The best way to obtain this reduced aging effect, whether you are a professional athlete or not, is to do at least 30 minutes of aerobic activity per day for 5 days a week. Doing sports you enjoy and that challenge you would be great, such as golf, tennis and even basketball. Taking lessons will help you get better. Exercises such as yoga, tai chi, or weightlifting two hours a week will maintain strength and balance. And balance, as we age, is incredibly important.

An example of how balance impacts the elderly is exemplified by the story of Dave's grandmother, Blanche, who lived long enough and stayed present long enough, both mentally and physically, to become more than the typical grandmother; as he grew into adulthood, Dave and Blanche became dear friends. They would get together at least once a week and often talked in between. Because they were so close, he could talk frankly to Blanche about her health and weight. Her choices weren't good ones. She was never one for doing much in the way of exercise or healthy eating and, like many of her generation, she smoked for most of her life. Living in a health-conscious way just wasn't a priority for her. He cajoled her but stopped short of nagging. Blanche made it clear she wasn't going to change, so there was no point in badgering her. She explained that she was the way she was, and she truly believed it was too late for her to do things differently.

As Blanche got older, she grew frail and eventually got very sick. She had to face a major operation and a drawn-out recovery, but she was strong and a fighter. As she struggled to recover, the falls hindered her. That time was scary for Blanche. She grew terrified of another setback but, try as she might, she simply couldn't keep her balance. After her third major fall she was readmitted to the hospital and died soon after. It's been more than 20 years, and she is still missed.

Nobody wants to fall and suffer the potentially horrific consequences. While there are many ways to stay in shape and reduce risk, there is no doubt that having good balance strength is imperative. Knowing this, there is a way that older individuals can maintain and even improve their balance!

To achieve positive results in balance; ballroom dancing is one of the most effective. The data bears this out. A study in Germany evaluated 62 healthy elderly volunteers between the ages of 61 and 94 living independently. For the study, they recruited two groups: one of long-time amateur dancers, dancing 16.5 years on average, and another group who had never danced. Several measures were used to test each group's posture and balance. Not surprisingly, the dancer's group was far superior to the non-dancer's group on all these measures.[7]

Those results were in people living independently. Would ballroom dance help those in assisted living to improve their posture and balance? Yes. Researchers looked at 59 residents of a nursing home. Half were assigned to the ballroom dance group. They danced for 30 minutes three times a week for three months, while the other half were controls asked not to exercise for the study period (but were promised they could join the dance group when the study was finished).

The groups were tested for balance and the number of falls experienced in the prior three months. For 12 weeks, the dancers participated in dancing sessions that started with a ten–minute warm-up followed by 30 minutes of the Foxtrot, Waltz, Rumba, Swing, Samba, or Bolero. Each session ended with a 10–minute relaxation period.

At the end of the study period, the dance group showed a 50% improvement in balance and a marked reduction in falls. The dancers also lost significant weight compared to the control group. Predictably, the control group enthusiastically joined the dancers at the end of the study.[8] It's been proven that Ballroom dancing is a safe activity that improves balance and reduces falls in the elderly.

Knowing how effective ballroom dancing is for people in a nursing home, you might wonder how well professional dancers do as they age. Do they have even better balance and better physical performance overall?

Another study in Germany addressed that question. They studied 49 healthy subjects. Eleven were competitive dancers and all, on average, 70 years of age. The study found the dancers performed better when it came to balance, posture, and reaction times compared to the healthy control group that did not dance.[9]

This is good news for all of us who are amateurs. It appears the act of learning and becoming a dancer (good, bad, or mediocre) is what provides the benefits. I not only have the evidence from the studies; I have firsthand experience of the benefits of balance from ballroom dance:

Here is my story.

I have always been a klutz. I used to trip and fall quite a bit. When I started ballroom dancing, I noticed my balance was terrible. I would tilt when I turned and I felt off-kilter. Initially, I could do one or two turns and feel okay. Any more than that, and I would feel nauseated and unsteady. I used to come home from my lessons and throw up. However, the more I danced, the less off-balance I felt. I am proud to share that now it no longer happens. I do not dread turning—now I enjoy it. I rarely trip when I am walking or climbing and descending stairs. I have excellent posture, and I feel very confident in my stance. My dancing has helped improve my balance, posture, and agility!

Physiologic Balance

Through dance, Dave and I have found balance not only in standing up solidly but physiologically. To excel at any exercise, the heart, gut, and brain must be balanced. We have seen that healthy systems on all three counts are essential for health and longevity. The same holds true for doing any kind of activity you want to do. It is not only dance, but golf, cycling, swimming, rowing, canoeing, running, hiking, and an assortment of other fun activities that require a certain level of health and fitness. That is why it is so essential for the foundation of your body to be as strong as the floor you are standing on. If that is not stable, you will definitely lose your balance and take a nasty tumble!

Just like Humpty Dumpty, you *all* fall down!

The Other Kind Of Balance

Looking at dance and what it requires, it can be seen as a metaphor for life.

First, you must be able to support your own weight and stand on your own.

Second, you need to be *flexible* when working with a partner. It is a give-and-take.

Third, you must be *willing* to lead, follow, or switch off. Two leaders or two followers just won't work.

Fourth, *communication* is key.

Fifth, when learning to dance, you must be *open* to learning a new language.

How does this apply to everyday living? When looking at life and work-life balance, the same principles apply.

Work-Life Balance

In my many talks over the years on this topic, I always find myself asking why people think there is such a thing as work-life balance? This implies we have total control over our lives. If you feel that, you're deluding yourself. Believe me, life has taught me that I have very little control. The key is to be *flexible*.

This was never clearer to me than when I was raising my children and trying to work full-time. When my kids got sick and couldn't attend school, I found a way to stay home from work. Rather than freak out and fret about it, I did things I usually couldn't do, like the laundry, picking up the day's toys, and spending precious one-on-one time hanging out with my ailing kiddo.

These principles are applicable to relationships, be they work or family. We must *be open* to learning about what is going to work for the partnership and, just as in partner dancing, the way we do this is with *communication*. It is also important to stand on our own and *carry our own weight* while being attuned to the other person/people and find a way to *work together* with cooperation, being willing to *lead and follow* as needed.

• • •

Life is a dance.

• • •

I learned to be flexible and roll with the punches. That is the only thing I can do. If you fight it, you get stressed, which isn't good for anyone. I suppose life itself is a dance, and learning the moves and what kind of dance you like is what works. So, do you want to search endlessly for work-life balance, OR would you rather dance? I know my choice. Dance, of course!

PART THREE

MAKE IT A PRACTICE

have given you many ideas on how to lead a fulfilling, peaceful and healthy life. Now you have a toolbox to do just that. However, what I cannot do is force you to use those tools. Your priority needs to be (here it comes, ladies…) YOU! Some people need to get to a certain level of desperation to make a positive change. Others can self-motivate before they get there. Here is an example of both.

Dana is 40 years old. At 5'5", she weighed in at over 200 pounds. When she married her husband, Jonah, at the age of 20, she weighed 125 pounds. After years of serially cheating on her, Jonah finally left her for a younger and thinner woman. He demeaned Dana and was downright nasty. She consoled herself by continuing to eat too much and move too little. One day, Dana decided she was tired of being tired and achy, as though someone else took over her body—she didn't even recognize herself in the mirror anymore—and she decided to just take a walk. She took herself outside and walked a block. She liked how that felt, and the next day walked two blocks. Before long, she was walking a mile a day. Then she found herself walking two miles a day and further increased her distance over the next few months.

Dana noticed her clothes were loose and after a month had lost at least 15 pounds. She felt happier and started eating healthier. She traded in the bagels for beans and the fruit juices for the real thing, whole fruits. The better she felt the longer she walked. The longer she walked, the more she wanted to do, including adding cycling to her regimen. After a year, she was feeling great, energized, free of achy joints, and was down to her normal weight of 125 pounds. She did so well that she joined a gym and started building muscle. She found a job, has new friends, and is on her way to a fulfilling and exceptional life.

As a footnote, her husband married the other woman and, ironically, they both found the weight Dana had lost.

Another patient of mine, Andrea, was very concerned about her health and highly motivated to change. She had a strong family history of heart disease and had just lost a close family member after they suffered a massive heart attack. Andrea was willing to do whatever it took to maximize her health. We evaluated her cholesterol, blood pressure, and exercise levels, and all were fine. But her TMAO levels (remember these are increased in some who eat red meat, farm-raised fish, and high-fat dairy) were sky high. She also had a very stressful job.

Andrea immediately cut out the red meat and other foods that cause elevated TMAO levels. She and her husband bought a small farm. She switched from a stressful desk job to one where she worked outside with lots of activity and animals she loved. Andrea felt fantastic. She slept better and was more fit than she ever thought possible. A year later, her TMAO levels, along with her stress levels, were normal. Andrea lost 15 pounds and increased her muscle mass. Her exercise tolerance doubled and she felt fantastic.

Both Dana and Andrea put themselves first and found a way to be their own best partner in health. Their methods of getting there were different, but the results were the same: both women shared the benefits of a healthier lifestyle and as a result were happier. They improved their well-being without completely overhauling their lives to make it happen. They took different approaches, but both made exercise, eating well, and managing their stress a priority and a practice. The realization that *you* (and only you) must be accountable for your health doesn't happen all at once like a lightning strike, but it is so important. I know it is not easy. Over almost 40 years of practice, I have heard about every excuse in the book. Here are some of the biggies.

• • •

I would eat better but healthy food is too expensive.

• • •

What is expensive are medical bills resulting from eating unhealthy food and the prescribed medications to treat the consequences of a poor diet. Healthy eating, with fresh vegetables and fruits, is more affordable than you think. Regardless of where you live, you can grow your own produce. There are kits for doing it inside and communal gardens for outside. Most food banks these days carry healthy produce.

I can't exercise. I don't have time. Most people watch television—they have time for that. You CAN exercise while you are watching. Walk in place, pedal a stationary bike, or get a treadmill. There are plenty of affordable, used equipment options out there. (I found a treadmill for under $200, and it works great). Take a break at work. Walk outside. You can just do 10 minutes at a time.

I can't take care of myself. I am too busy. Here is a fact. You cannot take care of anyone else if you are dead and gone. Ask for help and take a five-minute break from all the stressors and stressful people in your life. Take a short walk in nature. It really doesn't take much. Even sitting in a quiet place for 5 minutes away from the usual noise of your life can be enough to give yourself a peaceful time out.

The world is stressing me out. How can I relax and be happy? Guess what! You don't have to watch the news! Switch to the Discovery Channel instead. Or better yet, have a screen-free week every once in a while. Dr. Andrew Weil, the integrative medicine guru, suggests a "news fast". It is tough to do if you are a news junkie. However, I have done it, and it is very helpful. Take the news app off your phone. You can always put it back later. Watch a funny movie instead of CNN. The truth is, you can't do anything about world events. So, it is OK to take some time out to be uninformed and tune in to your own life and what is going on within you.

Being healthy is TOO Expensive. I disagree. Taking a walk in the park, joining a faith-based institution or a community group, planting a garden, and riding a bike to the store rather than taking a car—all are low-cost (or no-cost) alternatives to expensive gyms and gym equipment. Ballroom dance lessons are generally affordable when you learn with a group. And you will find that they are an inexpensive, healthy alternative for an evening of fun for the whole family. And rope in your friends! Going for a walk-and-talk with a friend is exercise without feeling like exercise—and it doesn't cost a penny.

"No Excuses: Make *You* A Daily Priority"

In the chapters to come, you will realize the power you have to find and consistently maintain a healthy practice to fine-tune your eating and exercise regimen, as well as handle the many stressors you may have in your life. First, what you put into your body is essential. Healthy, whole foods will help you feel and look good inside and out. Exercise will give your heart, brain, and gut a healthy edge. I have some easy tips anyone can follow, no sweat. And stress is something we all deal with. There are great ways to limit it and help you cope. The best part of what I propose is that they are not that hard to do. I give you small, palatable steps.

The key is consistency. Eating one healthy meal every three days won't cut it. Nor will getting in just one workout a week if you're sedentary for the rest of it. Small regular and consistent practices can make all the difference. This has been borne out in study after study. Mini workouts throughout the day are as good as one long workout.

Consistently making healthy choices about food will also make the difference. Over time you will realize how much better you feel and connect the healthy diet with how you feel. When this happens, you will be able to maintain this practice for life.

There is more! You can do a great one-hour workout in the morning, but if you sit all day, you negate the positive effects. Aim for at least 30 minutes of exercise daily and strive to make moving a "constant" in your life. Find something you like to do and can continue on a regular basis.

What is great about all this is that eating well, moving your body, and easing your mind, don't have to cost you a pretty penny. We'll explore how in the chapters to come.

Life is too short to spend it going from the doctor's office to the pharmacy and to be in pain (emotionally, physically, or both) and feel unwell. Our medical system is broken, and I am not sure that being on the disease treadmill will bring you even a step closer to wellness. You must take charge. One step at a time; tiny steps are OK. Just do it. Start with eating healthy and exercising. I will outline what sort of eating and exercise plan you might want to adopt. Spoiler alert! You are going to like both.

CHAPTER NINE

EAT TO YOUR HEALTH

The Blue Zones And The Mediterranian Diet

I love a good story, especially about learning. Most people will remember the story and, thus, the message that comes with it. So, I start this chapter with one of my favorites; an example of someone who finds a way to partner with himself and takes control of his health and well-being. The story of Stamatis Moraitis was told initially by Dan Buettner, author of *Blue Zones*, and it's a fascinating tale.[1]

As I wrote about earlier, in 2010, Dan Buettner, a National Geographics Fellow and best-selling author, found the five cultures around the world with the highest concentration of people living healthfully to 100 years or older: Okinawa, Japan; Sardinia, Italy; Nicoya, Costa Rica; Ikaria, Greece; and Loma Linda, California. Buettner used a blue pen to circle each region on the map in blue, which is how they came to be known as "Blue Zones." Stamatis Moraitis became an esteemed Blue Zone resident.[2]

Mr. Moraitis was an army veteran originally from Ikaria, Greece. He came to the US in 1943 to treat an arm injury he sustained during the war and found his way to Boynton Beach, Florida, where he met his wife and put down roots. In 1976, then in his mid-60s, Moraitis started to have shortness of breath. He went to his doctor and was diagnosed with lung cancer. His diagnosis was confirmed by multiple doctors, who all agreed Moraitis had about nine months to live. Treatment would buy him a little time but, instead, Moraitis returned to Ikaria to be buried alongside his ancestors. He figured he would also save money on a funeral since burial is cheaper in Ikaria.

He and his wife moved in with his parents, who lived on a small vineyard. The island is only 255 square miles and is rocky and rich with wild landscapes and beautiful beaches. It is also steeped in family traditions and vineyards that produce wine linked to some of the Ikarians' secrets to longevity.

When he moved to the island his health was failing and he was bedridden. His wife and mother cared for him, and he gradually recovered a small bit of strength. It was enough to allow him to get outside and enjoy the scenery and the fresh air.

Once he was up and ambulatory, he made his way to church on Sundays. His friends realized he had returned and came to visit. Every afternoon, he talked with them and drank some local wine. Over the 6 months that followed, things shifted for him. He felt stronger and good enough to plant vegetables, still expecting to be dead and gone when they were harvested. He thought it would be nice for his wife to have fresh vegetables after he passed.

Time came and went and Moraitis didn't die. He felt stronger. He was able to eat the vegetables he grew. He worked in his family vineyard, took naps, walked to the local tavern, and played dominoes with his friends. He thrived, and the cancer was no longer detected.

When Dan Buettner visited Mr. Moraitis in Ikaria, he asked if he could explain what had happened to the doctors who diagnosed him. He said he had tried, but when he returned to the US for a visit, all those doctors had retired and passed away. Mr. Moraitis lived to be 97 (102 by his own account).

Mr. Moraitis followed the Mediterranean diet. I believe it was the bedrock of his healthy transformation which, of course, was also accompanied by healthy lifestyle changes. This diet has been studied intensely and found to have significant benefits for health, happiness, and longevity. It is the one I recommend. As our Greek friend found out, food is medicine. If you choose correctly, it can be the best medicine for what ails you![3]

What is the Mediterranean diet? First, it is a pattern of eating rather than a diet. It includes vegetables, fruits, nuts, legumes (beans), seeds, and fish. It utilizes extra virgin olive oil and minimal dairy and red meat.

Basically, you eat like a Greek! Those who eat this way avoid processed foods, refined carbohydrates, sugar, and unhealthy fats. They do drink red wine in moderation. Why must you think about eating this way? There are many good reasons.

It reduces the risk of heart disease. We know that heart disease is the number one killer of men and women in the US, and multiple studies show the Mediterranean diet is a great way to eat for your heart. A 2013 study followed 7,000 men and women in Spain with type 2 diabetes who were at high risk for heart disease. Those who ate a Mediterranean-style diet with extra-virgin olive oil or nuts had a 30% lower chance of cardiac events.[4]

It reduces the risk of stroke in women. A study reported in 2018 observed a group of over 23,000 men and women between 40 and 77 who lived in the UK. The closer a woman followed the Mediterranean diet, the lower her risk of stroke—reduced by 20%. It did not have the same reduction effect in men.[5]

The diet may prevent dementia. A review published in 2016 found that sticking to this type of eating was associated with improved cognition and a lower conversion to Alzheimer's disease. A small study published in 2018 examined the brain scans of 70 people with signs of dementia. Those who scored low regarding the Mediterranean diet had more beta-amyloid deposits seen in Alzheimer's disease and two years later had even greater increases in deposits than those following the Mediterranean diet.[6]

If you want to lose weight, this can help. Analyzing the Spain study, I found that those following the Mediterranean diet had a smaller waist circumference and lost more weight than those who did not. Most people do not use calorie restriction with this eating pattern, but you will find a more dramatic weight loss if you do. Reaching your ideal weight is essential for overall health.[7]

You can live a longer life. A 2016 study from the European Heart Journal evaluated 15,000 people with heart disease from 39 countries. Those who followed the Mediterranean diet were less likely to have a stroke, heart attack, or die than those who did not.[8]

Eat this way and keep type 2 diabetes away! A group of 418 people between 55 and 80 without diabetes were studied. Those who followed the Mediterranean diet had a 52% lower risk for type 2 diabetes in a four-year follow-up period.[9] The diet improved blood sugar control in another study that reviewed 20 randomized clinical trials.[10]

This diet is anti-inflammatory. People with rheumatoid arthritis may benefit. This diet is rich in omega-3 fatty acids found to have an effect against inflammation in autoimmune diseases.[11]

What about cancer? It reduces the risk! As we saw with Mr. Moraitis, it made a difference. Granted, it wasn't just the diet that saved his life; but it was a significant contributor. A meta-analysis of 83 studies published in 2017 found that diet may reduce the risk of breast and colorectal cancer.[12] Another study showed women who ate a Mediterranean diet with extra-virgin olive oil had a 62% lower risk of breast cancer than those in the control group eating a low-fat diet.[13]

The Mediterranean diet can help with depression. A study published in 2018 analyzed 41 observational studies. The diet was associated with a 33% lower risk of depression when compared to a diet rich in processed meats, sugar, and trans-fat.[14]

The Mediterranean style of eating, at its core, is just healthy eating. It is all about whole foods, lean protein, healthy grains, avoiding processed meats and sugars, and using olive oil. So, come on! What's not to love about this diet? The beauty is you really don't need to count calories. Just pay attention to the quality of the food you put into your body.

As to healthy eating, there is something more you can do. We now have ways to see genetically how you process different medications and if they will work for you—and we can do the same thing for food. (Seriously, this is cool.) These tests assess how you metabolize certain foods and whether or not they will be a problem for you. Utilizing how your genes code for enzymes utilized for food metabolism they can also determine food allergies and certain sensitivities. For information on the most up-to-date tests, you can check out my website: triunemed.com.

Most tests can be done with a cheek swab and usually cost under $100 and can be purchased online. It will tell you if you are a slow metabolizer of carbs and/or fat, meaning you hold on to them and the calories they contain. It can tell you if you have or are prone to lactose intolerance. It can even tell you if you genetically have celiac. There are many other things it can tell you in addition to your best eating plan as a unique individual.

This test helped explain why I gained weight on the Atkins diet, the low-fat diet, and every other kind of ridiculous diet I ever tried; it also showed that if I stick to lean protein and vegetables, legumes and fruit, and whole grains, I can maintain a healthy weight. As you might have guessed, I am a slow metabolizer of fats and carbohydrates!

So now you know the key. Stick with healthy foods and know your genetics. For weight loss, the Mediterranean-style diet with calorie restriction is effective. Remember from the Longevity chapter one more useful eating tip to take from the Blue Zones: stop eating when you are 80 percent full. This is called Hara Hachi Bu. As I mentioned earlier, my husband thinks he is a healthy eater (he's NOT) and does not follow this philosophy. He eats until he is stuffed. As you may recall, his nickname is Hara Hachi Bu Bu, or as I call him, Bu Bu baby.

As we age, it is essential to keep in mind that weight gain is not inevitable. Even though most women think this is true, studies dispute this. It can be combated by making muscle.

Muscles can be increased easily with strength training and healthy dietary changes. Over many years of practice, I have seen that any change is difficult, even when that change can make a difference in overall health and well-being, it is hard for people to do.

Let me give you an example.

A patient, Jill, had rheumatoid arthritis. She was overweight and eating foods high in carbohydrates. Worse, she was addicted to Coca-Cola (the real thing!). When she begged me for a "natural" solution to her inflammatory condition, I explained the importance of an anti-inflammatory diet. She balked a little, but when I told her she had to stop drinking Coke, she just couldn't do it. It took extreme pain and desperation for her to finally give it up. And it helped. Her pain diminished and she could back off on her medication.

To switch to an anti-inflammatory diet, such as the Mediterranean diet, many of my patients struggle with adhering to it consistently. They assume that a day or two of healthy eating is enough; they don't get that it is a full-time deal! Fitness and health are crucial to getting the most out of your life and reclaiming wellness.

While we may look at certain foods as guilty pleasures, there is no reason to feel guilty anymore. In fact, some have tremendous health benefits. First up is my favorite!

COFFEE

Some specific foods and drinks have gotten a bad rap. Coffee is one of them. I must come clean and confess, I am hooked on it. I started drinking coffee after school in junior high with my mom and her friends. I felt so grown up as I regaled them with my tales of teenage woe and explained how I was never going back to school.

Obviously, I went back to school and kept drinking coffee. I have kept up with studies about this tasty brew since I have a vested interest in making sure it is okay for me to drink. There was a bit of a scare in 1981 when an article in the *New England Journal of Medicine* described an increased risk of pancreatic cancer associated with coffee drinking. It turns out the study was biased; the researchers matched the patients with cancer to control patients in the hospital for gastrointestinal problems. Those patients were told NOT to drink coffee even though many had been regular coffee drinkers, making it look like coffee was a factor in pancreatic cancer.[15] Fortunately, it is not. Since that time, many studies have looked at coffee and health. The benefits are many. Let's start at the top and work our way down.

The Brain

The most impressive effects of coffee are seen in the brain. Many of us find we need it to get going and prepare for the day. Of course, there is the ritual of drinking that first cup, but most importantly, it snaps us into focus. It has many other benefits beyond the "alertness" factor, particularly regarding neurologic disease. Coffee has been associated with a lower risk of Parkinson's disease. However, the protective effect was only with caffeinated coffee. Those who drink it are anywhere from 32- 60% less likely to develop the disease. It has also been found to improve motor function in those who have Parkinson's.[16]

Coffee also has a protective effect against Alzheimer's disease. The results of a large, long-term study known as the Cardiovascular Risk Factors, Aging, and Dementia (CAIDE) study found coffee drinkers had a 65% decreased risk of developing the disease.[17]

Coffee has been associated with a decreased risk of depression in women. For those who drank four or more cups a day, their risk of depression was reduced by 20%. A study at Harvard found those who drink two to four cups a day decrease their risk of suicide by 50%.[18] Why is coffee so effective? It increases our sensitivity to insulin, which may account for its positive effect on the brain.

Coffee drinkers are also able to focus when tired. After drinking a cup their reaction times, reasoning ability, and attention improve.[19] A combination of 11 studies found two-to-six cups a day was associated with a lower risk of stroke, about 20% compared to non-drinkers.[20]

Multiple sclerosis is a disease that affects 2.3 million people worldwide. An analysis of two case-control studies at Johns Hopkins University found a link between coffee consumption and MS. The researchers found participants who did not drink coffee in the year before the onset of symptoms were 1.5 times more likely to develop MS when compared to those who drank four cups of coffee a day. In this case, it appears caffeine is neuroprotective.[21]

Finally, the extensive Nurses' Health Study found women who consumed about six cups of coffee per day had a 21% decreased risk of developing tinnitus or ringing in the ears.[22]

Coffee is remarkable, and not just because I am hooked on it. It is the most popular drink in the WORLD, beating out tea. And the smell of coffee is the most common scent recognized in the US. How often does something this good not only make you feel better but keep you healthier (for the most part) as well? Rarely!

The Heart of the Matter

Although coffee can increase blood pressure when used sporadically and can cause the heart to race if one overindulges, researchers have found moderate, long-term coffee consumption of three to five cups a day lowers the risk of heart disease. This is probably due to the phytochemicals in coffee that reduce inflammation, the process that contributes to heart disease.

The Pancreas and Liver (The Gut)

Drinking six to seven cups of either caffeinated or decaffeinated coffee per day was found to reduce the risk of developing type 2 diabetes by 23-50%. Controlled studies have found that with each cup's consumption, the risk decreases by 7% up to five cups per day.[23]

Coffee decreases the risk of alcohol-related cirrhosis by up to 80% in those who drink four or more cups a day. It also reduces the risk in those with nonalcoholic fatty liver disease.[24]

Cancer Prevention

Drinking two cups of coffee daily reduces liver cancer risk by 40%.[25] Four to five cups a day reduces the risk of endometrial cancer by 20%.[26] It reduces the risk of lung cancer in those who smoke.[27] It may also reduce the risk of melanoma and basal cell cancers of the skin.[28]

A study compared 5000 people with colorectal cancer to 4,000 people without cancer. They found that those who drank two and a half cups of coffee per day had a 50% lower risk of colorectal cancer than those who did not drink coffee. Interestingly, it did not matter whether it was caffeinated or decaffeinated.[29]

Death Reduction(!)

Drinking coffee significantly reduces the risk of premature death by 20% in men and 26% in women.[30]

In Summary

Why is coffee so beneficial? It is probably due to the fact it is packed with antioxidants that keep us healthy. However, over-consumption can carry a few side effects to consider.

Aside from the potential cardiac issues mentioned above, the other downside to coffee is what it may do to your sleep if you drink it near bedtime. The other potential problem for regular drinkers is what happens if you stop. You will get a whopping headache. I make sure that never happens!

I would be remiss if I didn't remind you that while coffee has no calories, the calories can undoubtedly add up when you drink fancy coffee. A 20-ounce Mocha Frappuccino at Starbucks is 500 calories and has an astounding 79 grams of sugar. Finally, drip-filtered coffee is fine if you prefer to brew it at home. Coffee contains oils known as terpenes, which, if left in the brew, can raise LDL or "bad" cholesterol levels. The old-fashioned percolator coffee and the new-fashioned French press coffee make unfiltered coffee that may increase cholesterol levels. You might want to drink these types of coffee in moderation if cholesterol is an issue for you.

<u>CHOCOLATE</u>

Another one of my favorites, chocolate, has a deep and "rich" history. It goes back as far as 1900 BC in Mesoamerica. The Aztecs thought the cacao seeds were a gift from the gods. They believed it was an aphrodisiac and gave strength when consumed. For those of us in modern times, chocolate is revered for its taste, avoided due to its calories, and has been described as a guilty pleasure.

However, chocolate has been touted as a healthy food for the last several years. Chocolate contains the following:

- **Tryptophan**: a precursor to serotonin—naturally occurring chemicals that give us a sense of well-being

- **Caffeine**—a stimulant

- **Xanthine**—increases wakefulness

- **Theobromine**—a stimulant that increases blood flow and acts as a cough suppressant

- **Anandamide**—activates pleasure receptors in the brain

- **Phenylethylamine**—stimulates the release of dopamine, associated with feelings of pleasure

- **Flavanols**—plant or phytonutrients which act as powerful antioxidants that boost blood flow and act as a mild analgesic (i.e., pain reliever)

So, considering those qualities, is chocolate healthy? I say, yes! If eaten in moderation and in its pure form, the benefits make it a worthwhile treat. Let's start at the top again.

The Brain

Research at Harvard Medical School found seniors who drank two cups of hot cocoa per day for a month had improved blood flow of the brain and memory. It only worked with chocolate that contained high levels of antioxidants, otherwise known as dark chocolate.[31]

A Canadian study of over 44,000 people found those who ate chocolate were 22% less likely to suffer a stroke than those who did not. They were also 46% less likely to die as a result.[32] Chocolate also makes us feel good. It boosts endorphins and can create a similar effect to cannabis, but in a small way, because to make a real psychotropic impact, an average size person would have to eat 25 pounds. So, it may perk us up and make us happy due to the taste, texture, and overall experience.[33]

The Heart

Chocolate lowers the risk of developing heart disease by one-third of those who eat it regularly. In a study of 21,000 people from Norfolk, England that took place over 11 years of those who were in the top level of chocolate consumption, 12% developed cardiovascular disease compared to 17.4% who did not eat chocolate.[34]

A study of 470 elderly men found cocoa reduced the risk of cardiovascular death by 50% over 15 years.[35] Another study revealed eating chocolate five times a week lowered the risk of disease by 57%.[36] Yet another study found eating chocolate two or more times a week decreased the risk of calcified plaque in the arteries by 32%.[37]

Chocolate improves some of the risk factors for cardiovascular disease. The flavanols in dark chocolate stimulate the lining of blood vessels to relax, reducing blood pressure. Cocoa powder decreases LDL cholesterol in men and increases their HDL, or "good" cholesterol.[38]

The Skin

The flavanols in chocolate can protect against sun damage to the skin. In a study of 30 people, the time required to develop redness doubled after eating one-third of a two-ounce dark chocolate bar every day for 12 weeks.[39]

As If Chocolate Isn't Wonderful Enough

I have a tip for you: If you are in a movie, concert, or play and feel like you must cough, eat a piece of chocolate. I mentioned earlier that chocolate contains theobromine which acts as a cough suppressant. Taking a small square of dark chocolate and letting it melt on your tongue will stop your cough for about an hour. Keep some in your purse or pocket and give it a try the next time you must fight the urge.

In Summary

Chocolate in moderation is healthy. Eating a small square (1.5 oz.) with 70% or higher organic cocoa is important. The healing power is in the cocoa content.

LEMON BALM

Lemon balm can be considered food. It is also a fantastic treatment, so I just had to write about it for all of you cold sore sufferers. This is an excellent remedy to know about!

Ninety percent of Americans experience at least one cold sore in their lifetime. Forty percent have recurring infections. That is why a natural, inexpensive remedy would be a wonderful thing to have.[34] The herpes virus is responsible for causing cold sores *and* genital herpes. Generally, herpes virus 1 (HSV 1) causes cold sores, and herpes virus 2 (HSV 2) causes genital herpes.

Lemon balm, also known as *Melissa Officinalis,* is a great natural treatment for these viruses. The plant is easy to grow outside and can also grow inside. There are properties of the plant that explain its therapeutic effect. The leaves contain plant substances called tannins and terpenes that give the plant its antiviral effects. They also contain eugenol, which helps with pain and discomfort and kills bacteria.

Studies have shown topical lemon balm cream and ointments can heal cold sores. In one study of 66 people, lemon balm cream was applied, and patients experienced a significant decrease in redness and swelling after two days. Unfortunately, the cream did not affect the scabbing and discomfort.[40]

A series of impressive studies in Germany showed when lemon balm was used to treat a *first-time* infection of HSV 1, not a single recurrence was found. In addition, it reduced the healing time of both genital and oral herpes.[41]

How Can Lemon Balm Be Used?

Lemon balm can be found in ointments and creams, but soaking a cotton ball in lemon balm extract and dabbing it on the cold sore can also be very effective. Lemon balm tea can be used as a facial or body wash, or soak. Lemon balm soft gels can be taken orally. Preparations are relatively inexpensive, and if you want to be even more natural, you can grow the plant in your garden and make your own teas and extracts.

When To Use Lemon Balm?

For those plagued with cold sores, I recommend patients apply lemon balm nightly to their lips to prevent them. It feels good, works well, and keeps the lips from getting chapped. I suggest using the cream or ointment four to five times a day for outbreaks. For genital herpes, put the extract or tea in a bath and soak. It will be soothing at the very least, and many people find it helps with the intensity and duration of symptoms. It is worth a try, and fortunately, there have been no reported side effects.

MAGICAL MEDICINAL MUSHROOMS

Whenever I mention mushrooms to my patients, they start to giggle as they remember the psychedelic mushrooms of the '60s. But the mushrooms I talk about are medicinal. They are the same ones used in cooking, but I recommend the concentrated capsules for my purposes. Mushrooms are classified as vegetables, but they are not really plants. They are fungi. And they are amazing!

Many mushrooms can be used to detoxify contaminated environments. They have enzymes that break down plant fiber. These enzymes also reduce hydrocarbons and other manufactured toxins. Once they have finished their job, the pollutants can be used as fertilizer. And guess what else! What mushrooms do for the environment they also do for the body; they are excellent detoxifiers.

They also feed the microbiome discussed earlier, acting as prebiotics. As we explained, prebiotics are defined as nondigestible food components that promote the growth of beneficial microorganisms in the intestines. Asparagus, onions, and leeks are good examples (not to be confused with probiotics, live microorganisms that, when administered in adequate amounts, confer a health benefit to the host).

Research has shown Reishi and Turkey Tail mushrooms boost the immune system, balance the microbiota, improve digestion, and help with weight loss.[42] Because mushrooms are such great detoxifiers, it is important that when you eat them or use them in a medicinal blend, they are organic and have been grown in a controlled environment. Otherwise, you may consume them with all the toxins they are breaking down. For that reason, I recommend a particular brand of medicinal mushrooms. It is called Host Defense by Paul Stamets, the "mushroom king." He has been studying mushrooms for decades and has perfected his blends. You can find out more about him and his mushrooms at fungi.com. His products are sold online and at health food stores.

I recommend mushrooms to my patients for a whole host of reasons. Several varieties include Turkey Tail, Reishi, Maitake, Shiitake, Cordyceps, and Lion's Mane, and I'll briefly describe the benefits of each. If you want them all and then some, there is a blend of 17 mushrooms called MyCommunity, available commercially.

Reishi

The use of this mushroom goes back centuries. It was called the "Mushroom of Immortality." It has many positive effects, including immune-enhancing properties. It is also helpful in cancer treatments, disrupts viral illness, inhibits bacteria, and improves liver function. It has been found to lower blood pressure, improve allergies, act as an anti-inflammatory, and help to reduce stress and insomnia. This mushroom can calm tension, which is why some say it can extend life.[43]

Maitake

This mushroom is often called "The Hen of the Woods" because that is what it looks like. Its beneficial effects are numerous. In Asia, it is traditionally used to treat diabetes and high blood pressure. However, it may help with many other problems, one of which is improving fertility in those with polycystic ovarian syndrome. These women have difficulty getting pregnant due to hormonal issues.[44]

There are medications available to help; however, mushrooms are nutritious and without side effects. They can be used alone or to augment medical treatment. The maitake mushroom has an anti-tumor effect in bone marrow tumor colony formation and reduces the toxicity of some chemotherapeutic agents. It enhances immune activity against bladder cancer cells and reduces inflammation in inflammatory bowel disease. In a small group of cancer patients, the Maitake mushroom was found to induce tumor regression and it improved symptoms in half the patients.[44]

Shiitake

Shiitake mushrooms are commonly seen on restaurant menus because they are so tasty, but they also have remarkable healing properties. They are rich in B vitamins, selenium, copper, zinc, manganese, and vitamin D. They are an excellent source of iron that is easy for the body to access.

As to overall health effects, they reduce the risk of cardiovascular disease by protecting blood vessels. These mushrooms block harmful molecules from binding to the vessels and causing them damage. This cellular injury is responsible for atherosclerosis, otherwise known as the hardening of the arteries, which increases the risk of a heart attack. In addition, they also have antiviral and anticancer properties.[45]

Cordyceps

Cordyceps is a weird little fungus. It grows on caterpillars in the Himalayan Mountains. It has been used as a tonic in Chinese medicine to improve energy, found to improve blood flow, and helps you to breathe by opening your airways. It prevents bacterial and viral infections, reduces cholesterol, and increases sperm production in quantity and quality.

I was introduced to this mushroom in capsule form while training with Dr. Andrew Weil. I was shocked at the energy-producing effect it had on me, so I often recommend it to my patients. It is a great energy booster in the afternoon when people tend to get sleepy and does not interfere with sleep at night.

Turkey Tail

This mushroom is found all over the Pacific Coast of the United States. It lives on fallen hardwood trees and branches. It's so named because it looks just like a turkey tail. I recommend this mushroom to all my cancer patients or those with a family history of cancer. Studies first done in Japan and now in the United States have found that when used in combination with chemotherapy, it enhances the therapeutic effect. It also reduces the side effects of treatment. It is beneficial in treating breast, cervical, lung, esophageal, skin, and stomach cancers.[46] Studies are ongoing by the National Institutes of Health.

In addition to the above, Turkey Tail mushrooms have strong antiviral properties against viruses known to cause cancer. The two it's known to fight are the Human Papilloma Virus which causes cervical cancer, and the Hepatitis C virus, which causes liver cancer. The same study suggested it may inhibit HIV as well.[46]

To understand the potential power of these mushrooms, I'll tell you about a patient of mine. The story is quite remarkable.

Fifteen years ago, Helen, a 58-year-old woman, came to see me at my clinic. She had been diagnosed by biopsy with a rare skin cancer, Merkel cell carcinoma. It is a neuroendocrine tumor (stemming from the nerve and hormone system). Deviously, it appeared as a painless red bump on her left index finger which grew quickly and deeply. As you can imagine, Helen was pretty upset ("freaked out" were her words) when she found out. Due to scheduling and insurance issues, she and her doctor planned to have the whole tumor removed a month later at the University of Washington. I prescribed four capsules of the Host Defense Stamets 7 blend (containing Royal Sun Blaze, Cordyceps, Reishi, Maitake, Lion's Mane, Chaga, and Mesima) in the morning and four more Lion's Mane capsules in the evening before meals because she also had back pain, and Lion's Mane is known to help with nerve problems. She took them faithfully for a month, had her tumor removed and all seemed to have gone well. A month later, I received a call from her surgeon who wanted to know what I had done for her before the surgery. I told him I had started her on the mushrooms. He told me that between the time of the biopsy and the tumor removal, all the cancer cells had died. He believed the mushrooms had something to do with the tumor cell death. Helen continues to take her mushroom capsules and has remained in remission for fifteen years!

Lion's Mane

Lion's mane looks just like its name and is delicious and nutritious. When sautéed, it tastes like lobster and contains 20% protein.

Lion's Mane mushrooms used in the treatment of Merkel cell carcinoma continues to be explored. Merkel cell is a difficult tumor to treat, and one of the big challenges of this cancer is it has often spread by the time it is discovered. The medicinal mushroom Lion's Mane has proven effective treatment for some patients.[47] It certainly has been for my patient. After remaining cancer free on the mushroom capsules for fifteen years, Helen is convinced they've saved her life. For other patients with this kind of tumor, there is no harm in using it. There are no side effects, and it is considered a healthy food.

Lion's Mane mushrooms also protect the nervous system. There are studies in rats showing when the main nerve in the foot of the animal is crushed, it grows back when the rat is treated with the mushrooms.[48]

Lion's Mane has also been found to help with mild cognitive impairment. In a study reported in 2009, 30 subjects with Alzheimer's disease were given Lion's Mane capsules of 250mg three times a day for 16 weeks. Compared to the placebo, those given the mushrooms improved significantly. Four weeks after the study ended, they deteriorated. The mushrooms only worked to improve their memory while they were taking them.

Finally, yet another study, found those who ate Lion's Mane cookies versus those who ate cookies without it showed less anxiety and depression, and they were able to concentrate better![49]

One last food deserves an honorable mention: the magical fruit (and we know why that is…).

BEANS

What would you think if I told you there was a food that provided all of the following?

- Tons of fiber
- Lots of protein
- Keeps you at a healthy weight
- Promotes heart health
- Good for diabetes control
- A wonderful source of iron
- Provides magnesium
- Full of potassium.

I think it looks like great food—and it is! I am talking about BEANS. Beans have gotten a bad rap lately, largely due to the keto and paleo folks who eschew beans because they are high in carbs. However, when you look at beans from the perspective of the Blue Zones, you will find that all centenarians have a diet rich in beans. Beans are legumes in the family of vegetables with lentils, peas, chickpeas, and peanuts. They are good for us for all of the above reasons. They can be a bit of a problem when it comes to gas. However, a little bit of Beano before eating them and it won't be an issue!

Or, as my husband, the GI doctor, says, just enjoy your farts!

Finally,

When considering a healthy lifestyle, you might want to avoid being so restrictive. Many diets may not meet your long-term nutritional needs. Adhering to a keto diet where most vegetables and fruit are restricted or forbidden may cause you to miss out on critical micro-nutrients such as selenium, magnesium, phosphorus, and vitamins B and C. These are important for a healthy body.[50]

The paleo diet, where carbohydrates are severely restricted along with dairy, can result in calcium and vitamin D deficiencies.[51] Frankly, any restrictive diet gets boring and expensive and becomes nutritionally deleterious.

CONCLUSION

Hopefully, you have found a healthy, delicious way to eat from our description of the Mediterranean-style diet and fun foods you can eat. If you are someone who eats entirely differently from this, (for instance, you are a red and processed meat eater and/or used to eating packaged foods) you can switch over. You do not have to do it all at once. Start gradually. For example, what about reducing your red meat consumption from five times a week to once a week and slowly decreasing it to once a month? If you aren't used to eating vegetables, experiment and see which ones you like best. Cooking them in an air fryer helps to make them even tastier. Switch cooking oils to healthy oils. Start *somewhere* and then make small changes on a weekly or even monthly basis. You can do it, and you will see that you feel healthier over time. This incremental approach also works for exercise.

CHAPTER TEN

ONE CANNOT BE HEALTHY WITH HEALTHY EATING ALONE

• • •

Why do we need to move?

• • •

– MOVEMENT 101 –

There are so many reasons for doing it. When you sit, your big muscles are not using sugar. This can cause your blood sugar levels to rise. This in turn triggers the release of insulin, the hormone that regulates sugar. Over time, this causes the body to lose sensitivity to insulin. This results in inflammation leading to fatty plaques building on your arteries, increasing your risk of stroke and heart attack and a reduction in the diversity of the gut microbiome. There are many studies that support this phenomenon.

When 2,600 people aged 60 and older were studied and followed for 9 years, those who sat for 3 hours a day vs. those who sat for 7 hours a day were 33% less likely to die of heart disease during that period.[1]

It didn't take much activity to make a big difference

When 8,000 people were studied over 10 years, those who did light activity for 30 minutes a day instead of sitting had a 17% lower risk of dying during that period compared to the "sitters." The 30 minutes did not have to be consecutive.[2]

When 5,600 women were followed for 5 years, if they reduced their sedentary time by one hour a day, there was a 26% lower risk of heart disease. Again, the hour did not have to be reduced all at once, it could be incremental throughout the day. Short bursts of movement interrupting sedentary behavior was all it took.[3]

Exercise: Do It The Blue Zone Way

As people get older, they tend to think they no longer need to exercise. It turns out that just one out of four people between 65 and 74 exercises regularly. They worry that they are too out-of-shape, too tired, or too old for exercise with a sense that decline is inevitable. They feel it will be of no benefit. Furthermore, the prospect of intense exercise is overwhelming. You will see that anyone can and must exercise and that high-intensity exercise is not absolutely required for healthy aging.

Here is what I mean. For general fitness, a study of 78,500 people living in the UK followed those who wore a fitness tracker 24 hours a day for 7 days a week. They were on average 61 years old.

This study showed that up to 10,000 steps a day were associated with a reduced risk of cancer, heart disease and mortality for those with an average age of 60 years, for up to a seven-year follow-up period.

There was no minimum threshold for the benefits. People just needed to move. The UK study found that 9,800 steps per day could reduce dementia by 50% and just 3,800 steps per day could lower it by 25%.[4]

The best way to understand this concept of simply moving for fitness is to take you to the Blue Zones. The place where Stamatis Moraitis lived in Greece is one of them.

What Is A Blue Zone?

As I explained earlier, in 2010 Dan Buettner, a National Geographics Fellow and best-selling author, found five cultures around the world with the highest concentration of people living healthfully to 100 years or older. On the map, he circled them in blue, hence the name, "Blue Zones." The five original Blue Zones are Okinawa, Japan; Sardinia, Italy; Nicoya, Costa Rica; Ikaria, Greece; and Loma Linda, California.

These "zones" have certain qualities in common. Some of these include many things I have already mentioned, such as eating until you are 80% full, a plant-centric diet, and drinking wine in moderation. In addition, these groups have a community they belong to, have a higher purpose, and put family first. For exercise, they do not go to a gym; they move naturally. They incorporate movement as a natural part of life. That is what Mr. Moraitis did. They walk to the store, and garden, and explore nature.

This form of exercise is valuable. Even fidgeting is helpful. This is called ***non-exercise activity thermogenesis or NEAT***, the energy we utilize for everything we do other than sleeping, eating or sports activities. By moving all day long, people can get high "NEAT" scores. When this type of energy is *not* expended, our weight as well as inflammation in our body can rise. What this means is that small movements throughout the day make a difference.

You undoubtedly have heard that sitting is the new smoking, and this is why, for those of you who have been doing a lot of sitting…it is time to get up and move…even fidget.

Researchers checked the inflammatory marker c-reactive protein, triglycerides, and blood sugar increases in those who achieved NEAT compared to those who did not. This lack of activity can cause problems quickly.[5]

A study published by the American Diabetes Association showed that inactivity for just one day can cause cell processes to fail. This lowers good cholesterol (HDL).[6]

People in the blue zones have higher levels of NEAT on a regular basis. They walk to their friends' and neighbors' homes; they perform physical tasks and have regular exercise routines such as tai chi and yoga.

How Much Is Enough?

A total of two and a half hours of standing and light walking around the house or office is an adequate amount. Standing up for five minutes after every thirty minutes of sitting will make a difference.

Some other ideas include:

- A sit-to-stand desk.

- Walk after each meal.

- Walk to a coworker's office or desk instead of calling or emailing.

- Set your phone for a 30-second stretch and stand up for 5 minutes.

- Walk around your house when talking on the phone or watching TV.

- Take the stairs when you can.

- Walk an hour every day.

- Find an activity you like such as swim, run, ride a bike, or dance, and try to do it daily.

These activities provide a powerful strategy for exercise.

Furthermore, as we get older, we need to keep our muscles healthy. The best way to do that is with strength training.

We know that aging is associated with physiologic and functional decline which can lead to falls, disability, and frailty. It is a fact that aging leads to muscle loss. However, to prevent this, strength training 2 to 3 days per week is the answer. It builds muscle strength and muscle mass and maintains bone density. It is also good for preventing heart disease, type 2 diabetes, and arthritis.

I have trouble motivating myself, so I have a trainer I work with two days a week. I admit, I do not like it, but I do it. I know how important it is for my strength and vitality. I also use stretchy bands at home. I keep them in my family room and use them while watching movies or TV.

You don't need a trainer if you can self-motivate. Carry your groceries, find yoga exercises that utilize body weight, consult with a physical therapist to show you how to do this on your own, and then do it! The goal is to make exercise a natural part of your life, something you do every day that is easy and fun to do.

Tale Of Two Women

I just explained how the Blue Zone's method of movement works. To truly understand it here are the stories of two women; one who exercised her whole life and the other who claimed to be "allergic" to exercise.

Jane, born in 1930, was active her entire life. Her father died when she was young, so her mother raised her alone. She did a lot of chores around the house to help her mom. She also did all kinds of fun activities. She played tennis and went to sleep-over camp in the summers where she excelled in water sports. Her activity never stopped. She went to college and got married. She had children and was busy with them hiking, swimming, ice skating, skiing, and playing outdoor games. Once the kids grew up, she continued to play tennis and hike. In addition, she ate a plant-based diet with lean protein. She is still moving, she never stops. She is almost 94 years old and healthy and active. She is a force to be reckoned with indeed.

Joan, born in 1929, grew up with a single mother as well. Thanks to wealthy grandparents, she was afforded private schools, went to college, and got married. She hired nannies for her children. She was involved in teaching and all kinds of political activities. She had no time for exercise and was not active at home. She lived in an apartment in a major city and rode the elevator. She ate a diet rich in fats and processed foods. At the age of 70, her memory started to slip. She was diagnosed with Alzheimer's disease. By the age of 78, her dementia was so severe that she forgot how to eat. She died shortly thereafter.

Both women were educated. Both had comfortable lives. One was and continues to be active, the other was not. Granted, genetics may be at play to some degree, but healthy eating and exercise were the most likely reasons that Jane is still going strong, and Joan is gone.

What About Exercise And Weight Loss?

Canadian research has found that eating healthy is great but to remain fit, exercise is also necessary. A healthy weight and a normal BMI are important. When exercise is added to healthy eating, the fat mass lowers, and muscle-burning calories rise. If you have trouble losing weight, exercise helps. Sometimes, decreasing calories alone may slow down metabolism, making weight loss difficult. When 5,000 people were studied on a 900-calorie-a-day diet, those who did not exercise lost weight far more slowly than those who exercised.[7]

They took ten diet-resistant people and matched them to 10 diet sensitive people. They participated in a six-week exercise program, matched on age, weight, and BMI. They were told to eat their normal diet.

They worked out 3 times a week. They walked on the treadmill for 30 minutes, weight lifted, and did core strength exercises. The exercise group who had been diet resistant decreased their fat mass, waist circumference and body fat in contrast to the non-exercising diet-resistant group.

Weight Loss as a Byproduct of Healthy Choices

As I have already established, exercise alone does not result in weight loss. It needs to be coupled with a healthy diet. If you want to lose weight, exercise is important to burn the healthy calories you consume.[8] Unfortunately, many people hate to exercise.

Centuries ago, people had to move for life. They had no choice. They needed to tend to their crops, walk to stores, etc. These days we have all the modern conveniences we need to sit and NOT move. Some people even go to extremes to avoid it. I have seen parents driving slowly while following their children on the track team go for a run. My neighbor rides his ATV or car to take his dogs for a walk. Just to be clear, they walk, and he drives. Who knows, in the future people may use drones or robots so they don't even have to go outside to run their kids and animals.

Sadly, only half of adult Americans meet the minimal guidelines for adequate exercise. These are at least 30 minutes of moderate-intensity activity (fast walking counts) daily. It does not have to be accomplished all at once. Ten to 15-minute increments work. A quarter of American adults devote *no* free time to physical activity. They are completely sedentary. That is scary.[9]

You have one body. It is important to take care of it and find an activity that you can do consistently. If you don't use it, you'll lose it. Your muscles atrophy quickly with disuse. When my mom had a cast removed after she had broken her wrist at 40, her muscle on the broken arm had dwindled down and looked so small compared to the other arm, after just six weeks. The flip side is that after regular, consistent exercises, her arm size was normal again after another six weeks.

Think about what happens to your body if you sit around and become a couch potato for that long! If you have been sedentary and have lost muscle mass, have no fear, muscles can be built up again, just like my mother's arm. A physical therapist or trainer can show you what to do.

You need muscle to feel good and to have a healthy metabolism. It burns more calories than fat. It will help you maintain a healthy weight.

You don't have to look like a supermodel or have washboard abs. What I am talking about is being fit and arriving at a healthy weight so that you feel good. The byproduct is you look good inside and out, and that's what it's all about!

The key is to find something fun you like to do which coincidentally happens to burn calories. *Dancing (for me at least) is that activity.* It is fun and it helps with weight loss among many other benefits.

A study took 60 overweight Japanese women who participated in a weight loss program that encompassed diet and exercise for three months. The subjects were divided into two groups who either did aerobic dance or jogging and/or cycling. Both groups lost around seven pounds and about 6% of their body fat. Both forms of exercise worked. This study illustrates, at a minimum, dance is comparable to more traditional forms of exercise.[10]

What about the long-term? In 2012, a study of 100 overweight individuals between the ages of 40 and 70 were either given two-hour dance sessions with Latin and Standard Ballroom dancing twice weekly for six months or a self-selected sports activity that included cycling, aerobics, walking, or swimming. At three months, both groups had lost an average of about six pounds and had taken about 1.5 inches off their waistlines. This was maintained for six months. However, only the dance group was able to keep up the same high activity level after six months; the drop-out rate was much higher for the exercise group. That is because the dancers enjoyed themselves, so they kept on dancing.[11] AND THAT is the key!

Dance is fun and as a result, the benefits of weight loss and fitness have not been lost on the public. In fact, since 2014, dance has been the fastest-growing exercise and art form in Britain. More than 4.8 million people regularly attend community dance groups each year.[12]

How many calories are they burning while enjoying themselves? Slow ballroom dancing burns 207 calories an hour, and fast ballroom dancing can burn as many as 378 calories an hour. Swing burns 306 calories an hour and hip-hop burns the most at 465 calories an hour.[13]

Dance helps fight obesity along with a variety of other health problems. Whether you are overweight or just looking to stay at a healthy weight, it is time to get out there and dance!

The important thing about exercising, whether you are living in one of the Blue Zones or anywhere in the USA, is that you need to just do it. As we have seen, simply moving is what is most effective. When people do not exercise there are usually a host of excuses. Over my long career, I think I have heard them all. Here are some of the more common ones:

- **I can't afford a gym**. The truth is you don't need the gym. Most people who belong to a gym don't use it anyway, to the tune of 67%.[14] Go take a walk. Roaming around parks is free. Just walking is good for your body and moving every day is good for you.

- **My knees are bad.** Walking and exercise improve sore joints. If you have severe arthritis, consult with your doctor to find out just how much walking is good for you. I think you will find that gradually increasing the time and intensity of your exercise will be both safe and healing.

- **I have fibromyalgia**, exercise makes me hurt. People with fibromyalgia often hurt when they push too hard with exercise. For these patients, I recommend water exercise that can be done in a pool or hot tub. Just walking in place can make a big difference.

- **I hate doing weights.** If you don't like weights, get some yoga instruction, and use your body as weight. That works extremely well and (good news!) your weights are always with you!

- **I am too old to exercise.** This one always gets me. YOU ARE NEVER TOO OLD TO EXERCISE! Even if you do it in a chair or on a bed, you can do it. If you are severely debilitated, a physical therapist can help you figure out the best way to improve your activity level.

- **I am too fat to exercise.** Regardless of your weight, you have to start somewhere. If it is hard for you to move, just start small. A swimming pool may be the perfect place to start.

- **Exercise is boring.** For those who find walking boring, God invented audiobooks. It is amazing how far you can go when you are sucked into a good book. Walking with friends and having a good conversation also helps!

- **I don't have time to exercise.** Everyone has a half hour to spare. You can dance while you brush your teeth in the morning. You can take a break from your desk at work. You can walk outside, smell the roses, and come back inside. If you are really THAT busy, you can put a pedal bike under your desk or have a treadmill desk. You can move while you talk on the phone. Get inventive. It isn't that hard when you make it a priority and a practice.

There are oh so many more excuses I could go on to list for pages. I will spare you and tell you that exercise as a life practice is good for longevity and wellness and is a wonderful antidote for lifelong stress. Chronic stress can cause serious health problems. It is often discounted as just something we must deal with in life. However, it is important that it is not seen that way since stress can be deadly. Death may not happen suddenly but is more like death by a thousand cuts. I consider stress relief to be of major importance. In fact, I have signified its level as "the fifth" vital sign.

CHAPTER ELEVEN

THE FIFTH VITAL SIGN

There are four conventional vital signs in medicine. They include body temperature, blood pressure, pulse, and respiratory rate, the essentials that give nurses and doctors a sense of where your health is at the moment. I would like to propose a fifth vital sign. Something that will also give an idea of where you are both physically and emotionally. I call it "PCF." Otherwise known as **P**erceived **C**loseness to **F**reaking out. Here is the scale:

1. Calm and at peace

2. Slightly agitated—feeling that little niggle in your belly

3. Shaky and uneasy—pulse is starting to increase

4. Sweaty, breathing fast, and pacing nervously

5. Screaming, running around, curling up in a ball on the floor breathing in and out of a brown paper bag (or beating a couch with a foam bat)

Let me give you an example of what it looks like to get to number 5 on the PCF scale:

RIP Little Hamster

Many years ago, when my children were around 10 and 12, I had reached my limit. My son dyed his hair blue and left a huge ring of blue in the tub and sink (ala *The Cat in the Hat*). My other son threw a fit, we were all tripping over my husband's scattered shoes, and I was trying to work and take care of everything at home. I was freaking out! Someone suggested I take a foam bat, go into a room, shut the door and scream, and hit the couch. Great idea!

I went up to the kid's playroom and shut the door. In the room was our cute little hamster in a cage on one side of the room (Please note: nowhere near me or the bat). On the other was a futon. I picked up the bat and started beating the crap out of the mattress and screaming rather loudly. It felt great. I was at it for about 10 minutes. When I was done, I looked over at the hamster cage; there was the cute little aging hamster with his front paws clinging to the bars of the inside of the cage and he was dead. Frozen. I was shocked. Regardless, I did feel less stressed afterwards and realized just how angry and upset I must have been. I think my outpouring of emotion did him in. (Just as an aside, I had no idea that hamsters, especially old ones, can die of sudden death when exposed to noise and stress...of course, I do now!)

Some might criticize my issues and say they were "first-world" problems. That would be true. That does not mean they are any less stressful or upsetting. They were my reality and caused me stress and anxiety. I look at the hamster as a metaphor for my blood vessels and insides. I knew I needed to deal with them and deal with my issues to protect my health. I ultimately figured it out, which is partly responsible for why I wrote this book to help others, so many of whom are dealing with increasing levels of stress and anxiety.

Clearly, the PCF scale was designed with tongue in cheek. However, we are finding out just how important the impact of stress is on our lives. It takes its toll on every organ. The impact is especially hard on the brain, heart, and gut as I have outlined.

When stress becomes chronic it affects cognition reducing brain power. It eats away at the arteries of the body including the ones that feed the heart, the coronary arteries, and the gut becomes leaky and inefficient. The diversity of the microbiome is negatively affected and further increases the risk for cancer, dementia, heart disease, autoimmune disease, obesity, diabetes, and a variety of other conditions.

When there is an *acute* stress reaction it can be a good thing. If you are threatened, your body needs to get you ready to run and escape. That is where "Fight or Flight" comes from. It is a protective mechanism. If this reaction continues due to an ongoing perceived threat, that is when it becomes dangerous. What happens is that there is a continuous outpouring of stress hormones; the main ones being cortisol, adrenaline, and norepinephrine, which eat away at the body and deplete the adrenals...otherwise often known as "adrenal fatigue."

The ongoing perceived stress can be varied. For some, being in an abusive relationship can be like torture that becomes something a person just adapts to. A high-pressure, demanding job can do it. Family stress, financial stress, relationship stress; all these things can do it to you.

As to abusive relationships, finding a way out (not always easy) is essential. In other situations, you are often stuck. That is why it is important to deal with stress and find a way to reduce it. You can't necessarily change the circumstance. The only thing you can change is **YOU**.

In this book, we have given you the tools:

- **Eating healthy**

- **Exercising the NEAT way**

- **Dancing**

- **Finding nature by walking outside**

- **Meditating**

All these can help. Also helpful is stepping outside of yourself and finding gratitude and helping others. Both can be quite powerful. Does the expression of gratitude only help those who feel good to start with or can it help those who are stressed and having issues?

According to research, the answer is yes. A study of around 300 college students seeking mental health counseling was done by dividing them into three groups who all got counseling. The first group was instructed to write a letter of gratitude to another person for each week for three weeks. The second group was asked to write about their deepest thoughts and feelings regarding negative experiences. The third group did not have a writing activity. Those who wrote the letters had better mental health at 4 and 12 weeks compared to those who wrote about their feelings and those who didn't write at all.[1]

Another Important Question: How Does It Work?

The researchers analyzed the words used in the writing groups. They compared the percentage of positive and negative emotions expressed and the use of words in the first-person plural or what they called "we" words. Those in the gratitude group used a higher percentage of positive emotion and "we" words such as being thankful, appreciative, and grateful. Those with better mental health had more positive but significantly fewer negative words, and the lack of negativity correlated with mental health.

The gratitude letter writers were not required to send them. In fact, only 23% did. It was the act of writing the letter, not necessarily sending it, that was beneficial. Another interesting thing was that the benefits of writing the letters did not happen immediately; it took time. After one week of the study, there was no difference in mental health between the groups. However, the gratitude group started to improve significantly after 4 weeks and then even more at 12 weeks.

This study points out the value of gratitude and makes it even easier with the fact that the *writing* of the letter, not necessarily the sending of it, is what really matters. Finding ways to improve mental health is essential these days. Expressing gratitude is one way to do it. Write a letter today and keep doing it every week! You will be amazed at what can happen…in a good way!

What about paying it forward, especially regarding kindness and consideration?

When the pandemic hit and most people were isolated, I launched a postcard-writing campaign for my friends and family. I found funny cards and ones with interesting facts. I mailed over 100 of them. I heard back from many that they appreciated hearing from a friend while they were alone and lonely. Looking back, I realized that as much as it may have helped those who received them, it helped me more. It calmed me down. I felt like I was doing something valuable. We know from science that doing for others and gratitude is good for our health. Every religion espouses it, but few do it.

Paying it forward is an expression we hear often. It isn't about giving money or things; it is about doing good deeds and showing kindness in the care of others.

What is going on physically? Studies note that those who pay it forward also had a 23% lower cortisol level compared to the average population. Other studies show that random acts of kindness can improve feelings of self-esteem and self-worth. The other, very important thing is that it gets you out of your own mind. So, if you are stressed, you are removed from it by redirecting your focus. The other very cool thing is it has an immediate result!

Doing something kind for another person, no matter how big or small, leaves a positive impact on your mental health while also changing another person's day for the better. These actions go a long way. They cost nothing and bring a huge payoff when it comes to stress and disease.[2]

Taking The Concept Even Further

Another way to "pay it forward" is to become active in your community. This can be a good de-stressor and help you to feel good while helping others. The Blue Zones have this built into their lives. They have communities that support each other. In fact, not only does this happen in the five zones we spoke about, but it is happening all over the country with the Blue Zones Project.[3]

The Blue Zones Project is an initiative designed to change the way people experience the community around them. The goal is to create greater well-being, improved health outcomes, reduce medical costs, and build civic pride. The Blue Zones Project has come to many communities across the US. One of the great success stories is from the Beach Cities in California. The combined cities of Hermosa Beach, Manhattan Beach, and Redondo Beach prioritized policies to help their population make healthy choices easily and to be well. As a result, they have made huge inroads.

From 2010 to 2017 their residents' health improved:

There was a 25% drop in overweight adults.

36% decrease in smoking

5% drop in diabetes

An 8% increase in exercise

6% increase in produce consumption

4% drop in daily stress

4% increase in the number of people who **thrive.**

They did it by providing easier access to grocery stores, rather than having people feel the need to go to fast food restaurants. They installed bike lanes with direct access to work, stores, beaches, and parks. Other communities have added parks and have closed off streets to cars, making more walking streets. Most have encouraged community activities. We have seen this firsthand in the communities of Grants Pass and Klamath Falls here in Oregon. By helping each other, we find a way to thrive and find peace and happiness, together.[4]

THE DOCTOR'S NOTE

This book was written as a step-by-step guide to health and wellness. It has become increasingly important that we all become more accountable for our health. The medical system is broken. You really don't *want* to *have* to count on it. At this point, it is there for medical emergencies and the ordering of preventive health studies only. When it comes to your overall health, you are in the driver's seat. You are your best partner.

YOU ARE WORTH IT.

The good thing is that what you need to do to improve your health won't cost you a lot of money. However, it will take a major strength of will and willpower. My advice is to keep your eye on the prize and don't make too many changes all at once. It takes an average of two months to form a new habit. Studies show it takes 66 days, to be exact. So, be patient with yourself. [5]

Do one thing at a time. What you start with is your choice. But do it. Use your doctor for guidance when it comes to health measures. Get your recommended screenings and then find your way towards preventing disease and achieving wellness by eating healthy, exercising, relieving stress, and finding your way to feeling great. You don't have to slog your way through life and feel crappy. Rather, you can choose to dance and feel FABULOUS!

CONCLUSION

The message that has hopefully become crystal clear after reading this book is that YOU are your best partner in wellness. We have discussed and reiterated that lifestyle choices dictate how your one precious life flows. Unhealthy choices can maim and even kill you. Healthy choices will do more than keep you out of the hospital, they will improve your quality and quantity of life. Healthy lifestyle choices can be fun, doable and contrary to public opinion, don't suck!

For your brain, we have suggested fun activities such as meditation and ballroom dance, and turned you on to the power it contains, especially the mind-expanding power of learning.

For your brain and heart, we have suggested the yummy Mediterranean-style diet and NEAT exercise,

AND

For your brain, heart, and gut we have given you multiple tips on how to have a healthy microbiome. A healthy microbiome is the key to preventing acute and chronic diseases and can afford you a long and healthy life!

Whenever I decide to make a change, I set a goal. Usually, that goal is set at a reasonable distance in the future. I take small steps and keep going. The way I do that is by realizing that if I had started that change (for example) nine months earlier, I would already be done. By realizing that, I can keep on going. When I get to the goal, I think, "Look at that!"

If you are not choosing or maximizing healthy choices remember, if nothing changes, nothing changes. Get on the road to wellness and DO IT NOW! It doesn't matter how old you are or where you start out physically, you can make healthy strides no matter what. You just need to start. It can be difficult; change is tough for most of us.

Sometimes it can take a while, even years, for the message to get through. But I guarantee that no one has regretted making better, healthier choices. I doubt anyone looks back and says, "I'm sure I'd be in a better place if I never stopped eating donuts."

Or, "I'd be feeling so much better if I never started exercising."

The hard part is deciding to start. Remember, if you set your expectations too high, you are more likely to fail. Small changes are best.

Small Changes Make A Big Difference

The remarkable thing is that once you get started, the consistent small changes can yield big results. Making changes one at a time is often the best way to go.

We have seen:

By Losing just five pounds you can relieve tremendous pressure on sore knees.

By starting and maintaining a fun exercise program such as dance, it is possible to lower high blood pressure enough to be able to stop antihypertensive medications.

By walking each day and slowly increasing the distance covered, a person can lose weight that significantly adds up over a year. (See story on page 171)

By consistent ballroom dancing, mobility changes in Parkinson's disease can be slowed and even prevented.

By eating a delicious Mediterranean diet, you can prevent heart disease, Alzheimer's disease, depression, and a leaky gut.

Just think of what is possible if you make even more changes, like getting more sleep and cutting out artificial sweeteners! There are more rewards and fun once you start making your changes. You can track your success!

Technology For Good

I have talked about the evils of technology when the patient is left out of the equation. But, when you are your best partner in wellness, you can take full advantage of the technology available to you.

- For your vital signs, there are phone apps. You can check your blood pressure, oxygen levels, and pulse rate on your phone. The one I use is iCareHealth.

- You can do your own EKG rhythm strip using the Kardia app on your phone. I keep the little device that syncs up with the phone in my purse. If I feel palpitations, I check out my heart rhythm. It is quick and very helpful.

- Apple watches are getting very sophisticated. They give you blood pressure and EKG readings *and* provide body temperature readings.

- For sleep, my preference for a couple of years has been the Oura ring. It tells me how much REM and deep sleep I get and when I don't do as well as "it" thinks I must, it gives me tips on what to do to improve my sleep.

- There are even smart beds available that track your sleep and adjust if you need your head higher or need the mattress to firm up or even give you a massage. They tend to be quite expensive ($1000 to 9000+). Whether or not they live up to the hype remains to be seen.

Something important to keep in mind. I mentioned this in the beginning, and it bears repeating, especially now that you have the tools to make a difference in your life; 80% of chronic disease can be attributed to unhealthy lifestyle choices. By choosing a healthy diet, exercising, stress reduction, health preventive measures, and finding your passion and joy you can find your path to wellness.

We all must be accountable for our health. The key is to be informed and be smart about it. Find someone who can be your *partner* in wellness and guide you to become the healthiest person you can be. Enlisting an integrative medicine provider as a partner can make all the difference. If you can't find an integrative practitioner, at least find one who listens.

. . .

You can do it!

. . .

**Now, go forth and find your way
utilizing this guide to wellness.**

**You *can* do it. You *must* do it.
Your life depends on it.**

ABOUT THE AUTHOR

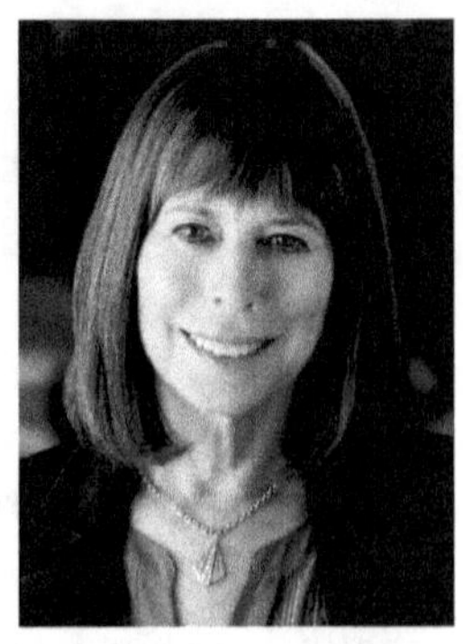

Dr. Robin Miller has gathered the knowledge, insights and information offered in this book over the course of 34 years of treating patients using the principles of integrative medicine and her personal experience.

Board certified in Internal Medicine, she trained with Andrew Weil as an Integrative Medicine Fellow at University of Arizona. She is currently Medical Director of Triune Integrative Medicine, a highly innovative, consultative integrative medicine company in Medford, Oregon. She serves as an Executive Advisory Board member for Sharecare, an interactive health and wellness website founded in conjunction with Oprah and Jeff Arnold (Creator of WebMD).

An established author (*The Smart Woman's Guide to Midlife and Beyond; Kids Ask the Doctor; Healed: Health and Wellness for the 21st Century;* and *Invisible or Invincible: Your Choice*), Robin is also a well-respected medical reporter and a regular correspondent for KOBI-TV NBC5, the NBC affiliate in Southern Oregon. She has produced the award-winning health series, "Is there a Doctor in the House," which is shown on the Wellness Channel nationwide. Her Health Tips are seen regularly on Triunemed.com and KOBI-TV NBC5. In addition, she writes a regular medical column for the Grants Pass Courier.

She lives in southern Oregon with her husband and trusty dog, Vegas. In her free time when she isn't dancing, she tends to the vineyard they have planted and developed together known as Peter William Vineyard.

ACKNOWLEDGMENTS

I would like to first acknowledge my co-author from *Healed: Health and Wellness for the 21st Century*, Dave Kahn. Without his encouragement and previous collaboration, I would not have attempted authoring a book. He has helped me to find my voice through writing as well as dance.

I thank my family for their support, my husband Peter, sons David and Brian and my beautiful dog Vegas who never left my side through the whole process.

Finally, I acknowledge all the people who helped me to write this book and put it together: Ann Maynard (editor) and Ginna and David Gordon (editors and designers). Thank you for all your encouragement, ideas, and support.

REFERENCES

Prologue

1. Vorghese,J. 2003

Introduction

1. Trimble, M 2018
2. CDC, 2022
3. Thimbleby, H. 2013
4. CDC, 1999
5. Cleveland Clinic, 2020

PART ONE:
SMARTS, HEARTS, AND FARTS

Chapter 1: The Brain

1. Smithers, L 2012
2. Hopkins, J. 2022
3. Farhangi, M 2020
4. Northwestern, 2019
5. National Geographic Kid, 2015
6. Ackerman, S 1992
7. Cleveland Clinic, 2020
8. Shoichet, C 2021
9. Qulilian, C. 2016
10. Fleischman, M 2008
11. CFI Team, 2019
12. Endocrine Society, 2022
13. Alzheimer's Association, 2022
14. Harvard, 2020
15. Hippius,H. 2003
16. Alzheimer's Society, 2022
17. Weeks, J 2016
18. Cutuli, D 2016
19. Zhang, Q 2020
20. Vargas-Soria, M 2021
21. Lemere, C 2010
22. Trafton, A 2016
23. Houser, K.
24. Weiler, M 2019
25. Van Dyck, 2022
26. Snowdon, D. 2003
27. Vorghese, J. 2003
28. Powers, R 2010
29. Kim, S. 2011
30. Erickson, K 2014
31. Parkinson's Foundation, 2022
32. American Parkinson Disease Association, 2022
33. Hopkins Medicine, 2022
34. NIH, 2022
35. Kwakye, G 2017
36. Parkinson's Disease Society, 2008
37. CDC,2019
38. Parkinson's Foundation, 2022
39. University of Alabama, 2022
40. Ray, F 2021

41. Earhart, G 2009

42. Duncan, R 2011

43. Brown, S 2008

44. YouTube, 2016

45. Xue, L 2020

46. CDC, 2021

47. CDC , 2022

48. Kenborg,L 2015

49. Hurt, C 1998

50. Teixeira, D 2022

51. Goderez, B 2019

Chapter 2: The Heart

1. Whelton,P. 2017

2. Marmic, P 2021

3. CDC, 2022

4. Fang, J 2019

5. Castaneda, R 2022

6. Palmer, S, 2009

7. Million Hearts, 2019

8. Corti, M 1997

9. Barger, S 2022

10. Heinza, Y 2017

11. Lassale, C 2018

12. Warren, T 2010

13. Golaszewski, N 2022

14. Prabhakaran, D 2017

15. Conrad, N, 2022

16. Raghavan, S 2019

17. Levine, G 2021

18. Emeasoba, E 2022

19. Blackwell, D 2018

20. Lakicevic, N. 2020

21. Thomson, B 2022

22. Vallance, J 2018

23. Cleveland Clinic, 2018

24. CDC, 2022

25. Hadanny, A 2020

26. Kyewoong, K 2020

Chapter 3: The Gut

1. Almario, C 2018

2. Gershon, 1999

3. Huang,T 2019

4. Liu, J 2022

5. Breit, S 2018

6. Canovan,C 2014

7. MedlinePlus, 2020

8. Gurjal, N, 2012

9. Al-Toma, A. 2019

10. Mahmud, N. 1999

11. Crohn's Colitis Foundation, 2020

12. Delvaux.M. 1997

13. Halland, M 2014

14. Chao, G 2014

15. Lee, H 2014

16. Gauschi-Ferre, M. 2021

17. Ursell, L 2012

18. Wan, M 2020

19. Zagursky, E 2015

20. Li, N 2019

21. Kulecka, M 2016

22. Monda, V 2017

23. Bleistein, A 2016

24. Siddiqui, M 2021

25. Evans, C 2014

26. Gershenson, G 2017

27. Gregor, M 2019

28. Debras, C 2022

29. Belkaid, Y 2014

30. Bander, A 2020

PART TWO:
STAY ALIVE AND THRIVE

1. Basmo, 2022

Chapter 4: Boost Your Brain

1. Medline, 2022

2. Wu, R 2019

3. Brennan, D 2019

4. Marisol, S. 2022

5. Lardone, A 2018

6. Nuwar, R 2012

7. Ireland, T 2014

8. Berbari, G 2018

9. Bates, C 2012

10. Luders, E 2009

11. Fleischman, M 2005

12. Fleishchman, M 2006

13. Vielle, R 2019

14. Dahl, C 2020

15. Grinberg, J 1997

16. Furman, 2022

17. Flexman, R 2021

18. Costandi, M 2018

19. NSC, 2022

20. NIH, 2022

21. Patel, AK. 2022

22. Pacheko, D 2022

23. Mayo Clinic, 2022

24. Sieburn, A 2012

25. Allen, K 2013

26. Novotney, A 2013

27. Bradt, J 2013

28. Maurier, R 2013

29. Kwan, M 2013

30. Rose, F. C 2010

31. Shaw, G 2022

32. Ashoori, A 2015

33. Jacobsen, J 2015

Chapter 5: Longevity

1. Nicita, M 2008

2. Stanford, 2021

3. Chopik, WJ

4. Haag, S. 2021

5. Reza, J.N. 2023

6. Science Learning Hub, 2011

7. Colen, BD, 2014

8. Goldman, B., 2021

9. Minhas, P.S. 2021

10. Zullo, JM 2019

11. Dai, S 2021

12. Chen, X

13. Dicorato, A. 2021

14. Armitage, H. 2020

15. Leslie, M 2000

16. Mineo, L 2017

17. Blue Zones, 2023

18. Yarnall, C 2011

Chapter 6: Improve Your Mood

1. NIH, 2022

2. Northwestern University, 2009

3. Ziegelstein, R 2023

4. Phillips, Q. 2021

5. Kandler, C 2019

6. Wan, L. 2018

7. Al-Harbi, KS. 2012

8. Shelton, R 2013

9. Legg, TJ 2019

10. PTSD Guidelines, 2017

11. IMDB, 2008

12. Limbana, T. 2020

13. Skolkovo Institute of Science and Technology, 2022

14. Chen, Y 2021

15. Khalili, P 2022

16. Seppälä, 2013

17. Ho, C. 2016

18. Institute of Medicine, 1998

19. Menon, V 2020

20. Jorde R 2008

21. Ding, J 2022

22. Gan, R 2008

23. Tanksanen, A 2008

24. Sarris, J 2012

25. Wani, A 2015

26. Penckofer, S 2017

27. NIH, 2017

28. Mayo, 2020

29. Duke, 1999

30. Hoffman, B 2011

31. Duke, 2000

32. Pinniger, R 2012

33. Schwarcz, J. 2017

34. Hoffman, K 2022

35. Statista, 2020

36. World Dance Sport, 2023

37. World Dance Sport/Fit through Dance 2023

38. GeneSight, 2023

39. Panchai, N 2021

40. Yang, B 2019

41. Richards, T 2014

42. Knaus, B 2012

43. Ruhl, T 2022

44. Torres, L 2021

Chapter 7: SEX

1. Rutkowski, K 2014

2. APS, 2017

3. Sweet, L 2020

4. Frappier, J 2013

5. Hendrick, B 2010

6. Smith, B 2023

7. Liu,Hu 2016

8. Liu, H 2016

9. Mozes, A 2016

10. Iffgd,2023

11. Gu, Y 2022

12. Bunis, D. 2018

13. Bote, J 2020

14. Stulberg, D 2008

15. Abraham, C 2023

16. Krause, M 2009

17. Medicine Magic, 2023

18. Dmitrovic, R 2013

19. W.K 2022

20. Editors, 2016

21. Bauer, M 2016

Chapter 8: Finding Balance

1. CDC, 2021

2. Seidler, R 2010

3. Horton, S. 2008

4. Peirce, D 2021

5. Averill, G 2018

6. Ben-Zur, 2002

7. Kattenstroth, J 2010

8. Gomes, E 2014

9. Woei, P 2015

PART THREE:
MAKE IT A PRACTICE

Chapter 9: Eat to your Health

1. Buettner, D 2012

2. Blue Zones, 2023

3. Hopkins, J 2023

4. Estruch, R 2013

5. Peterson, K.E. 2018

6. Hardman, R 2016

7. Barnard, N.D. 2020

8. Stewart, R 2016

9. Salas, J 2011

10. Ajala, C 2013

11. Schonenberger, K 2021

12. Morze, J 2021

13. Toledo, S,2015

14. Lassale, C 2019

15. MacMahon, B 1981

16. Hong, C 2020

17. Eskelinen, M2010

18. Dwyer, M 2013

19. Penetar, D 1994

20. Zhang, Y 2021

21. Hedstom, AK 2016

22. Glickman, J 2014

23. Muley, A 2012

24. Kennedy, O. 2021

25. Bravi, F 2013

26. Lafranconi, A 2017

27. Tang, N 2010

28. Whiteman, H 2015

29. Schmit, S 2016

30. Lopez, E 2008

31. Jaslow, R 2013

32. American Academy of Neurology, 2010

33. Australian Academy of Science, 2018

34. Grimmer, D 2015

35. Bujisse, B 2006

36. Yuan, S 2017

37. Djousse, L 2011

38. Mursu, J 2004

39. Williams, S 2009

40. Schnitzer, P 2008l

41. Garber, A 2021

42. Jayachardran, M 2017

43. Healthline, 2023

44. Wilson, D 2017

45. Begum, J 2022

46. Kubala, J 2018

47. Perez, A 2023

48. Wong, K 2011

49. Flynn, H 2023

50. Harvard, 2020

51. UC Davis, 2022

Chapter 10: One Cannot Be Healthy with Eating Alone

1. Henschel, B 2017

2. Stamatakis, E 2018

3. Harvard, 2020

4. Berman, R 2022

5. Wu, S 2014

6. Colberg, S 2016

7. Pileggi, C. 2022

8. Mayo Clinic, 2021

9. Harvard, 2019

10. Kwon, H 2017

11. Mangeri, F 2014

12. Leigh, S 2014

13. Burned Calories, 2023

14. Williams, B 2021

Chapter 11: The Fifth Vital Sign/ Doctor's Note

1. Brown, J 2017

2. Fewings, N 2019

3. Blue Zones, 2023

4. BCHD.org 2023

5. Clear, J. 2023

BIBLIOGRAPHY

Abraham, C. "Experiencing Vaginal Dryness? Here's What You Need to Know." www.ACOG.org 2023

Ackerman, S., English, P., Pinkney, J. "Discovering the Brain." *National Academies Press* (US). 1992

Ajala,O. "Systematic review and meta-analysis of different dietary approaches to the management of type 2 diabetes." *The American Journal of Clinical Nutrition*, Volume 97, (p 505-516) Issue 3, March 2013

Al-Harbi KS. "Treatment-resistant depression: therapeutic trends, challenges, and future directions. Patient Prefer Adherence." 6:369-88. Epub 2012

Allen, Kimberly A. "Music therapy in the NICU: is there evidence to support integration for procedural support?" *Advances in Neonatal Care:* official journal of the National Association of Neonatal Nurses vol. 13,5 (2013): 349-52.

Almario, C. V., Ballal, M. L., Chey, W. D., Nordstrom, C., Khanna, D., & Spiegel, M. R. Burden of Gastrointestinal Symptoms in the United States: Results of a Nationally Representative Survey of Over 71,000 Americans. *The American Journal of Gastroenterology*, (113(11), 1701. 2018

Al-Toma A, Volta U, Auricchio R, Castillejo G, Sanders D, Cellier C, Mulder CJ, Lundin KAE. "(ESsCD)guideline for coeliac disease and other gluten-related disorders." *European Society for the Study of Coeliac Disease United European Gastroenterol J.* 2019.

Alzheimer's Organization. "The patient journey inan era of new treatments." https://www.alz.org/media/documents/alzheimers-facts-and-figures.pdf. 2023.

Alzheimer Society. "The History Behind Alzheimer's Disease". https://alzheimer.ca/en/about-dementia/what-alzheimers-disease/history-behind-alzheimers-disease. 2023

American Academy of Neurology: American Academy of Neurology. "Can chocolate lower your risk of stroke?" *ScienceDaily*, 12 February 2010

APDA. "Death and Parkinson's Disease." https://www.apdaparkinson. org/article/death-parkinsons-disease/ 2023.

APS. APS https://www.psychologicalscience.org/news/releases/a-48-hour-sexual-afterglow-helps-to-bond-partners-over-time. html. 2017

Armitage, H. "Ageotypes' provide window into how individuals age." https://med.stanford.edu/news/all-news/2020/01/_ageotypes_-pro-vide-window-into-how-individuals-age--stanford-st.html. 2020

Ashoori, Aidin et al. "Effects of Auditory Rhythm and Music on Gait Disturbances in Parkinson's Disease." *Frontiers in Neurology* vol. 6 234. 2015

Australian Academy of Science: Can Chocolate Make You Happy? https://www.science.org.au/curious/people-medicine/can-choco-late-make-you-happy. 2018.

Averill, G. The Secret to Athletic Longevity Is Surprisingly Simple: https://www.outsideonline.com/health/training-performance/athletic-longevity-play-on-book. 2018.

Bander, A. Zahraa et al. "The Gut Microbiota and Inflammation: An Overview." *International Journal of Environmental Research and Public Health* vol. 17,20 7618. 19 Oct. 2020

Barger, S., Struve, G. "Association of Depression With 10-Year and Lifetime Cardiovascular Disease Risk Among US Adults, *National Health and Nutrition Examination Survey*, 2005–2018." CDC, Original Research. Vol. 19, 2022

Basmo. Is It Better to Read or Listen to a Book? https://basmo.app/listening-to-audiobooks-vs-reading. 2022

Bates, C. "Is this the world's happiest man? Brain scans reveal French monk has 'abnormally large capacity' for joy - thanks to medita-tion." https://www.dailymail.co.uk/health/article-2225634/Is-worlds-happiest-man-Brain-scans-reveal-French-monk-abnormally-large-capacity-joy-meditation.html 2012

Bauer, Michael et al. "Let's talk about sex: older people's views on the recognition of sexuality and sexual health in the health-care setting." *Health Expectations*: an international journal of public participation in health care and health policy vol. 19,6 1237-1250: 2016

BCHD. "Healthy Communities" https://www.bchd.org/healthpolicy 2023

Begum, J "Shiitake Mushrooms: Health Benefits, Nutrition, and Uses." WebMD, www.webmd.com/diet/health-benefits-shiitake-mushrooms 2022

Belkaid, Y., Hand. T. "Role of the microbiota in immunity and inflammation." Cell vol. 157,1: 121-41. 2014

Ben-Zur, H. "Coping, affect and aging: the roles of mastery and self-esteem." *Personality and Individual Differences*. 32:2: 357-372. 2002

Berbari,G. "Why Meditation Can Actually Make You A Happier Person, According To Science." https://www.elitedaily.com/p/why-meditation-makes-you-happy-according-to-science-8333117 2018

Berman, R. "10,000 Steps vs. Power Walking: Are they equally beneficial?" https://www.medicalnewstoday.com/articles/10000-steps-vs-power-walking-are-they-equally-beneficial. 2022

Blackwell, D., Clarke, T. State Variation in Meeting the 2008 Federal Guidelines for Both Aerobic and Muscle-strengthening Activities Through Leisure-time Physical Activity Among Adults Aged 18–64: United States, 2010–2015 *National Health Statistics Reports* Number 112-28, 2018

Bleistein, A. "Could Your Workout Impact Your Gut Health? Yes— And Here's Why " https://www.linkedin.com/pulse/could-your-workout-impact-gut-health-yesand-heres-why-abby-bleistein/ 2016

Blue Zones: "Live Better and Longer." https://www.bluezones.com/, https://www.bluezones.com/2023

Bote, J. "How much sex should couples have? Here's what experts say." https://www.usatoday.com/story/news/health/2020/02/07/ how-much-sex-should-couples-have/4680968002. 2020

Bradt J, Dileo C, Shim M. Music interventions for preoperative anxiety. *Cochrane Database Syst Rev.* 2013 Jun 6 (6);2013

Bravi, F., Bosetti C., Tavani, A, et. al. "Coffee Reduces Risk for Hepatocellular Carcinoma: an Updated Meta-analysis" *CGHI Journal.* Vol 11:11 p1413-1421 2013

Breit, S., Kupferberg, A., Rogler, G. et.al. "Vagus Nerve as Modulator of the Brain–Gut Axis in Psychiatric and Inflammatory Disorders." *Frontiers in Psychology*, 13 Vol 9-2018

Brennan, D. "Learning After 60." https://www.webmd.com/healthy-aging/learning-after-60. *WebMD.* 2021

Brown, S. "So You Think You Can Dance? PET Scans Reveal Your Brain's Inner Choreography. Recent brain-imaging studies reveal some of the complex neural choreography behind our ability to dance." *Scientific American*.299,1: 2008

Brown, J., Wong, J. New research is starting to explore how gratitude works to improve our mental health." *The Greater Good Magazine*.https://greatergood.berkeley.edu/article/item/how_ gratitude_changes_you_and_your_brain. 2017

Buettner, D. "The Island Where People Forget to Die. https://www. nytimes.com/2012/10/28/magazine/the-island-where-people-forget-to-die.html 2012

Bunis, G.,, Yuanyuan et al. "Gut and Vaginal Microbiomes in PCOS: Implications for Women's Health." *Frontiers in Endocrinology* vol. 13 808508. 23 Feb. 2022

Burned. "How many calories do you burn with Dancing?" https:// burned-calories.com/sport/dancing. 2023

Canavan, C. et al. "The epidemiology of irritable bowel syndrome." *Clinical Epidemiology* vol. 6 71-80. 4 Feb. 2014, doi:10.2147/CLEP. S40245

Castenada, R., Urban, A. "Ornish Diet." https://health.usnews.com/ best-diet/ornish-diet . 2023

CDC. "Life Expectancy in the U.S. Dropped for the Second Year in a Row in 2021." https://www.cdc.gov/nchs/pressroom/nchs_press_releases/2022/20220831.htm. 2022

CDC: "Obesity epidemic increases dramatically in the United States: CDC director calls for national prevention effort." https://www.cdc.gov/media/pressrel/r991026.htm. 1999

CDC. "Facts about Falls." https://www.cdc.gov/falls/facts.html 2023

CDC. " Traumatic Injury and Concussion." https://www.cdc.gov/traumaticbraininjury/index.html. 2021

CDC. 1918 Pandemic. https://www.cdc.gov/flu/pandemic-resources/1918-pandemic-h1n1.html. 2021

CDC. Heart Disease Facts. https://www.cdc.gov/heartdisease/facts.htm 2021

CDC. "Stroke Symptoms." https://www.cdc.gov/stroke/signs_symptoms.htm 2022

CFI. "Meditation: Boost Your Memory and IQ." https://corporatefinanceinstitute.com/resources/elearning/meditation-boost-your-memory-and-iq/2023

Chao, Guan-Qun, and Shuo Zhang. "Effectiveness of acupuncture to treat irritable bowel syndrome: a meta-analysis." *World Journal of Gastroenterology* vol. 20,7: 1871-7. 2014

Chen, Y.,Silan, G., Yunbo, C. et al. : Six-month follow-up of gut microbiota richness in patients with COVID-19. *GUT.* Jan;71(1):222-225. 2021.

Chopik, W. Bremmer, R, Johnson, D et. al. "Age Differences in Age Perceptions and Developmental Transitions." *Frontiers in Psychology*, 01 February: Vol 9Sec. Personality and Social Psychology. 2018

Clear, J. "How Long Does it Actually Take to Form a New Habit? (Backed by Science) https://jamesclear.com/new-habit. 2023.

Cleveland Clinic. "5 Healthy Habits That Prevent Chronic Disease. And how to make healthy lifestyle habits permanent." https://health.clevelandclinic.org/5-healthy-habits-that-prevent-chronic-disease/ 2020.

Cleveland Clinic Newsroom. "Cleveland Clinic Studies Reveal Role of Red Meat in Gut Bacteria, Heart Disease Development." https://newsroom.clevelandclinic.org/2018/12/10/cleveland-clinic-studies-reveal-role-of-red-meat-in-gut-bacteria-heart-disease-development/ 2018.

Cleveland Clinic. " Amazing Facts You Didn't Know About Your Brain." https://health.clevelandclinic.org/brain-teasers-infographic/ 2020

Colberg, S., Sigal., "Physical Activity/Exercise and Diabetes: A Position Statement of the American Diabetes Association." *Diabetes Care* 2016;39(11):2065–2079. 2016

Colen, BD Hope for Aging Brains, Skeletal Muscle Harvard Gazette. https://news.harvard.edu/gazette/story/2014/05/hope-for-aging-brains-C. 2014

Conrad, N., Verbeke, G.,Molenberghs et.al. "Autoimmune diseases and cardiovascular risk: A population-based study on 19 autoimmune diseases and 12 cardiovascular diseases in 22 million individuals in the UK. *The Lancet.* Vol 400:10354. 2022

Corti, M C et al. "Clarifying the direct relation between total cholesterol levels and death from coronary heart disease in older persons." *Annals of Internal Medicine* vol. 126,10: 753-60. doi:10.7326/0003-4819-126-10-199705150-00001. 1997

Costandi, M. "The Sleep Deprived Brain." The Dana Foundation. https://dana.org/article/the-sleep-deprived-brain/ 2018

Crohns & Colitis. "Colorectal Cancer Risk" https://www.crohnscolitisfoundation.org/science-and-professionals/education-resources/colorectal-cancer-risk-ibd. 2020

Cutili, D, Pagani, M, Caporali, P et. al."Effects of Omega-3 Fatty Acid Supplementation on Cognitive Functions and Neural Substrates: A Voxel-Based Morphometry Study in Aged Mice." *Frontiers in Aging Neurosci.* Vol 8: 2016

Dahl, C., Wilson, C., Davidson, R. The plasticity of well-being: A training-based framework for the cultivation of human flourishing. *PNAS.* 117(51). 2020

Dai, S., Qu, L., Li, J.,Chen, Y. "Toward a mechanistic understanding of DNA binding by forkhead transcription factors and its perturbation by pathogenic mutations." *Nucleic Acids Research*, Volume 49, Issue 18, 11 October 2021

Debras, C., Chazelas E., Sellem, L., Porcher, R. Artificial sweeteners and risk of cardiovascular diseases: results from the prospective NutriNet-Santé cohort. *BMJ* 378:2022

Delvaux, M et al. "Sexual abuse is more frequently reported by IBS patients than by patients with organic digestive diseases or controls. Results of a multicentre inquiry. French Club of Digestive Motility." *European journal of gastroenterology & hepatology* vol. 9,4 1997.

DiCorato, A. "Centenarians have a distinct microbiome that may help support longevity. Intestinal microbes in people aged 100 or over produce unique bile acids that might help keep infections at bay." *Broad Institute*. 2021.

Ding, J., Zhang, Y., "Associations of Dietary Vitamin C and E Intake with Depression. A Meta-Analysis of Observational Studies." *Front Nutr.* Vol. 9. 2022.

Djoussé, Luc et al. "Chocolate consumption is inversely associated with calcified atherosclerotic plaque in the coronary arteries: the NHLBI Family Heart Study." *Clinical Nutrition* (Edinburgh, Scotland) vol. 30,1: 38-43. 2011

Dmitrovic R, Kunselman AR, Legro RS. Sildenafil citrate in the treatment of pain in primary dysmenorrhea: a randomized controlled trial. *Hum Reprod.* 2013 Nov;28(11):2958-65. 2013.

Duke University. "Exercise May Be Just as Effective As Medication For Treating Major Depression." *ScienceDaily*. ScienceDaily, 27 October 1999. www.sciencedaily.com/releases/1999/10/991027071931.htm.

Duke Today. Study. "Exercise Has Long-Lasting Effect on Depression." 2022 https://today.duke.edu/2000/09/exercise922.html

Duncan, R., Earhart, G. *Randomized Controlled Trial of Community-Based Dancing to Modify Disease Progression in Parkinson Disease. Neurorehabilitation and Neural Repair.* 26(2): 132-43. 2011.

Dwyer, M. "Coffee drinking tied to lower risk of suicide." *Harvard Gazette*. 2013 https://news.harvard.edu/gazette/story/2013/07/drinking-coffee-may-reduce-risk-of-suicide-by-50/

Earhart, G M. "Dance as therapy for individuals with Parkinson disease." *European journal of Physical and Rehabilitation Medicine* vol. 45,2: 231-8. 2009.

Editors: https: Health Myth: Does the average man really think about sex every 7 seconds. GQ//www.gq.com/story/health-myth-does-the-average-man-really-think-about-sex-every-7-seconds. 2016.

Emeasoba, E. Ibeson, E. Nwosu, I. et. al. " Clnical Relevance of Nuclear Magnetic Resonance LipProfile." *Frontiers in Nuclear Medicine*. Sec. Radiopharmacy and Radiochemistry. Vol 2:2022.

Endocrine Society: "Brain Hormones." https://www.endocrine.org/patient-engagement/endocrine-library/hormones-and-endocrine-function/brain-hormones. 2022.

Erickson, Kirk I et al. "Physical activity, fitness, and gray matter volume." *Neurobiology of Aging* vol. 35 Suppl 2: S20-8: 2014.

Estruch, R., Ros, E., Salas-Salvado, J et. al. Primary Prevention of Cardiovascular Disease with a Mediterranean Diet. *New England Journal of Medicine*. 368:1279-1290. 2013.

Evans, C., LePard, K. J., Kwak, J. W., et.al. "Exercise Prevents Weight Gain and Alters the Gut Microbiota in a Mouse Model of High Fat Diet-Induced Obesity". *PLOS ONE*, 9(3), e92193. 2014.

Fang, J., Luncheon, C., Ayala, C. *MMWR Weekly*. 68(5);101–106. 2019

Farhangi, M. et al. "Gut microbiota-associated metabolite trimethylamine N-Oxide and the risk of stroke: a systematic review and dose-response meta-analysis." *Nutrition Journal* vol. 19,1 76. 30 Jul. 2020

Fennings, N. "7 Reasons Why You Should Pay It Forward For Your Mental Health. I Don't Mind." https://idontmind.com/journal/pay-it-forward-for-your-mental-health. 2019

Fleischman, M., Othmer, S. Case Study: "Improvements in IQ Score and Maintenance of Gains Following EEG Biofeedback with Mildly Developmentally Delayed Twins." *Journal of Neurotherapy*. 9(4): 35-46 2005

Flexman, R. "Lifelong Learning. A Key Weapon in Delaware's Fight Against Cognitive Decline." *Delaware Journal of Public Health* vol. 7,4 124-127. 27 Sep. 2021

Flynn, H. "Improving Memory Lions Mane Mushrooms May Double Neuron Growth" https://www.medicalnewstoday.com/articles/improving-memory-lions-mane-mushrooms-may-double-neuron-growth.2023

Frappier, Julie et al. "Energy expenditure during sexual activity in young healthy couples." PloS one vol. 8,10 e79342. 24 Oct. 2013

Fuhrman U. "History of Olli." 2023 https://www.furman.edu/osher-lifelong-learning-institute/who-we-are/history-of-olli/

Gan, R., et al. "Vitamin C deficiency in a university teaching hospital." *Journal of the American College of Nutrition* vol. 27,3: 428-33. 2008

Garber A, Barnard L, Pickrell C. Review of Whole Plant Extracts With Activity Against Herpes Simplex Viruses In Vitro and In Vivo. *Journal of Evidence-Based Integrative Medicine.* 26; 2021

GeneSight: https://genesight.com/2023

Gershenson, G. " A Brief and Bizarre History of Artificial Sweeteners." *Saveur.* 2017 https://www.saveur.com/artificial-sweeteners/

Gershon,M. *The Second Brain: A Groundbreaking New Understanding of Nervous Disorders of the Stomach and Intestine.* Harper Collins: November 17, 1999

Glicksman, Jordan T et al. "A prospective study of caffeine intake and risk of incident tinnitus." *The American Journal of Medicine* vol. 127,8: 739-43.2014

Goderez,B. " Treatment of Traumatic Brain Injury With Hyperbaric Oxygen Therapy." *Psychiatric Times*: 36:5. 2019

Goldman, B. "Study reveals immune driver of brain aging." *Stanford Medicine News.* https://med.stanford.edu/news/all-news/2021/01/study-reveals-immune-driver-of-brain-aging.html 2021

Gregor, M. "Not Sweet Nothings: Why Splenda and Stevia Can Make You Gain Weight." *Forks Over Knives.* 2019 https://www.forksoverknives.com/wellness/artificial-sweeteners-can-make-you-gain-weight

Grimmer, D. "Research on 21,000 Norfolk people leads scientists to link eating chocolate to lowered risk of heart disease and stroke." *Eastern Daily Press.* 2015

https://www.edp24.co.uk/news/health/20901286. research-21-000-norfolk-people-leads-scientists-link-eating-chocolate-lowered-risk-heart-disease-stroke/

Grinberg, J. "Ideas About a New Psychophysiology of Consciousness: The Syntergic Theory." *The Journal of Mind and Behavior.* 18:4. pp. 443-458 (16 pages) 1997

Golaszewski, N., LaCroix, A. Gordino, J. et. al. "Evaluation of Social Isolation, Loneliness, and Cardiovascular Disease Among Older Women in the US." *JAMA* 5(2) 2022

Gomes, E.,Gomes, R.,Cadir, A., et. al. "Postural balance and falls in elderly nursing home residents enrolled in a ballroom dancing program." *Archives of Gerontology and Geriatrics*: 59:2 2014

Guasch-Ferré, M, Willett, W.C. "The Mediterranean diet and health: a comprehensive overview." *Journal of Internal Medicine* vol. 290,3: 549-566.2021

Gu, Yuanyuan et al. "Gut and Vaginal Microbiomes in PCOS: Implications for Women's Health." *Frontiers in Endocrinology* vol. 13 808508. 23 Feb. 2022, doi:10.3389/fendo.2022.808508

Gujral, N., Freeman, H. J., & Thomson, A. B. (2012). Celiac disease: Prevalence, diagnosis, pathogenesis and treatment. World *Journal of Gastroenterology : WJG*, 18(42), 6036-6059. 2012

Haag,S. , Jylhävä, J., "Sex differences in biological aging with a focus on human studies." *eLife* vol. 10 e63425. 13 May. 2021

Hadanny, Amir et al. "Hyperbaric oxygen therapy improves neuro-cognitive functions of post-stroke patients - a retrospective analysis." *Restorative Neurology and Neuroscience* vol. 38,1: 93-107. 2020

Halland, A., Almazar, R., Atkinson, E., et. al." A case-control study of childhood trauma in the development of irritable bowel syndrome" *Neurogastroenterology & Motility.* Vol 26:7 2014

Hardiman, R., Kennedy, G., Macpherson, H., et. al. "Adherence to a Mediterranean-Style Diet and Effects on Cognition in Adults: A Qualitative Evaluation and Systemic Review of Longitudinal and Prospective Trials." *Front Nutr.*, Vol 3. 2016 https://www.frontiersin.org/articles/10.3389/fnut.2016.00022/full

Harvard. "Dementia incidence declined every decade for the past thirty years." Harvard News. 2020 //www.hsph.harvard.edu/news/press-releases/dementia-incidence-declined-every-decade-for-past-thirty-years/

Harvard. "Should You Try the Keto Diet?" Harvard Health. 2020 https://www.health.harvard.edu/staying-healthy/should-you-try-the-keto-diet

Harvard. "Why you should move-even just a little- throughout the day." 2020 https://www.health.harvard.edu/heart-health/why-you-should-move-even-just-a-little-throughout-the-day

Harvard. "Why we should exercise- and why we don't. 2019 "https://www.health.harvard.edu/newsletter_article/why-we-should-exercise-and-why-we-dont

Hedström, A K et al. "High consumption of coffee is associated with decreased multiple sclerosis risk; results from two independent studies." *Journal of Neurology, Neurosurgery, and Psychiatry* vol. 87,5: 454-60. 2016

Heianza, Y., et al. "Gut Microbiota Metabolites and Risk of Major Adverse Cardiovascular Disease Events and Death: A Systematic Review and Meta-Analysis of Prospective Studies." *Journal of the American Heart Association* vol. 6,7 e004947. 29 Jun. 2017

Hendrick, B.," More Sex Could Mean Less Heart Risk." 2010 https://www.webmd.com/heart-disease/news/20100121/more-sex-could-mean-less-heart-risk

Henschel, B., et al. "Time Spent Sitting as an Independent Risk Factor for Cardiovascular Disease." *American Journal of Lifestyle Medicine* vol. 14,2 204-215. 1 Sep. 2017

Hippius, H., Gabriele, N. "The discovery of Alzheimer's disease." *Dialogues in Clinical Neuroscience* vol. 5,1. 2003

Ho, C., et al. "Prevalence and Predictors of Low Vitamin B6 Status in Healthy Young Adult Women in Metro Vancouver." *Nutrients* vol. 8,9 538. 1 Sep. 2016

Hoffman, Benson M et al. "Exercise and pharmacotherapy in patients with major depression: one-year follow-up of the SMILE study." *Psychosomatic Medicine* vol. 73,2: 127-33. 2011

Hoffman. K., "41 New Fitness & Gym Membership Statistics [Infographic]" *Noogains*. 2022 https://www.noobgains.com/gym-membership-statistics/

Hong, Chien Tai et al. "The Effect of Caffeine on the Risk and Progression of Parkinson's Disease: A Meta-Analysis." *Nutrients* vol. 12,6 1860. 22 Jun. 2020

Hopkins. "The Genetic Link to Parkinson's Disease."2023 https://www.hopkinsmedicine.org/health/conditions-and-diseases/parkinsons-disease/the-genetic-link-to-parkinsons-disease

Hopkins. "Can your gut health affect your heart?" *Hopkins Health*. 2023. https://www.hopkinsmedicine.org/health/wellness-and-prevention/can-your-gut-health-affect-your-heart

Hopkins. "Take your diet to the Mediterranean." *Hopkins Health*. 2023. https://www.hopkinsmedicine.org/health/wellness-and-prevention/take-your-diet-to-the-mediterranean

Horton, S., Baker.,Schorer, J. "Expertise and aging: maintaining Skills through the lifespan." *European Review of Aging and Physical Activity*. Vol, p 89-96. 2008

Houser, K. "MIT is testing light and sound to combat Alzheimer's." *FreeThink*. 2022. https://www.freethink.com/health/gamma-waves-alzheimers

Huang, T., Lai, B., Du, L., Xu, Y., Ruan, M., & Hu, H. (2018). Current Understanding of Gut Microbiota in Mood Disorders: An Update of Human Studies. *Frontiers in Genetics*, 10. 2019

Hurt, C., Rice, R., McIntosh, G., et.al. "Rhythmic Auditory Stimulation in Gait Training for Patients with Traumatic Brain Injury." *Journal of Music Therapy*, 35:4, p 228-241. 1998

Iffgd. IBS in women. IBS Center.org: https://aboutibs.org/what-is-ibs/ibs-in-women. 2023

IMDB: https://www.imdb.com/title/tt0390521/characters/nm1041597 2023

Ireland, T. "What Does Mindfulness Meditation Do to Your Brain? As you read this, wiggle your toes. Feel the way they push against your shoes, and the weight your feet on the floor. Really think about what your feet feel like right now - their heaviness." *Scientific American*: Guest Blog 2014

Jacobsen, J., Stelzer, J., Fritz, T., et. al. "Why musical memory can be preserved in advanced Alzheimer's disease." *Brain*: Vol 138 (8) P 2438-2450. 2015

Jaslow, R. "Two cups of hot cocoa a day sharpen seniors' brains, study suggests." *Harvard News*. 2013 https://hms.harvard.edu/news/two-cups-hot-cocoa-day-sharpen-seniors-brains-study-suggests

Jayachandran, M. et al. "A Critical Review on Health Promoting Benefits of Edible Mushrooms through Gut Microbiota." *International Journal of Molecular Sciences* vol. 18,9 1934. 8 Sep. 2017

Jorde, R et al. "Effects of vitamin D supplementation on symptoms of depression in overweight and obese subjects: randomized double-blind trial." *Journal of Internal Medicine* vol. 264,6: 599-609. 2008

Kahili, P., Asbaghi, O.,Aghakhani, L., et. al. "The effects of folic acid supplementation on depression in adults: a systematic review and meta-analysis of randomized controlled trials" Nutrition & Food Science. 2023 https://www.emerald.com/insight/content/doi/10.1108/NFS-02-2022-0043/full/html

Kandler, Courtney E., Sherrell, L.. "Methylenetetrahydrofolate Reductase Screening in Treatment-Resistant Depression." Federal practitioner : for the health care professionals of the VA, DoD, and PHS vol. 36,5: 207-208.2019

Kattenstroth. J., Kolankoska, I., Kalisch, T. et. al. "Superior Sensory, Motor, and Cognitive Performance in Elderly Individuals with Multi-Year Dancing Activities." *Frontiers in Aging Neuroscience*: 2(31) 2010

Kenborg, Line et al. "Head injury and risk for Parkinson disease: results from a Danish case-control study." *Neurology* vol. 84,11: 1098-103.

Kennedy, O.J., Fallowfield, J.A., Poole, R. et al. All coffee types decrease the risk of adverse clinical outcomes in chronic liver disease: a UK Biobank study. *BMC Public Health* 21, 970. 2021

Kim, Se-Hong et al. "Effect of dance exercise on cognitive function in elderly patients with metabolic syndrome: a pilot study." *Journal of Sports Science & Medicine* vol. 10,4 671-8. 1 Dec. 2011

Knauss,B., "Overcoming Shyness and Social Anxieties Successfully combat social tensions by stepping out of character." *Psychology Today*. 2012. https://www.psychologytoday.com/us/blog/science-and-sensibility/201206/
overcoming-shyness-and-social-anxieties

Krause, Megan et al. "Local Effects of Vaginally Administered Estrogen Therapy: A Review." *Journal of Pelvic Medicine & Surgery* vol. 15,3: 105-114. 2009

Kubala, J. "5 Immune-Boosting Benefits of Turkey Tail Mushroom." Healthline 2018 https://www.healthline.com/nutrition/
turkey-tail-mushroom

Kulecka, Maria et al. "Prolonged transfer of feces from the lean mice modulates gut microbiota in obese mice." *Nutrition & Metabolism* vol. 13,1 57. 23 Aug. 2016

Kwakye, Gunnar F et al. "Disease-Toxicant Interactions in Parkinson's Disease Neuropathology." *Neurochemical Research* vol. 42,6: 1772-1786. 2017

Kwan, M., Soek Tian Seah, A. "Music therapy as a non-pharmacological adjunct to pain management: Experiences at an acute hospital in Singapore." Progress in Palliative Care . Vol 21(3). 2013

Kwon,N., Nam, S., Park, Y. e. al "Effect on 12-week Intensive Dietary and Exercise Program on Weight Reduction and Maintenance in Obese Women with Weight Cycling History." *Clinical Nutrition Research* 6(3):183 2017

Kyuwoong, K., Choi, C., Hwang, S., et.al. "Changes in exercise frequency and cardiovascular outcomes in older adults." *European Heart Journal*. Vol 41(15), pages 1490-1499. 2020

Lafranconi, Alessandra et al. "Coffee Decreases the Risk of Endometrial Cancer: A Dose-Response Meta-Analysis of Prospective Cohort Studies." *Nutrients* vol. 9,11 1223. 9 Nov. 2017

Lakicevic, N. et al. "Make Fitness Fun: Could Novelty Be the Key Determinant for Physical Activity Adherence?" *Frontiers in Psychology* vol. 11 577522. 15 Oct. 2020

Lardone, A. et al. "Mindfulness Meditation Is Related to Long-Lasting Changes in Hippocampal Functional Topology during Resting State: A Magnetoencephalography Study." *Neural Plasticity* vol. 2018

Lasalle C., Tzoulaki, J., Moons, K., et.al. "Separate and combined associations of obesity and metabolic health with coronary heart disease: a pan-European case-cohort analysis ." *European Heart Journal*, Volume 39, Issue 5, 01 February 2018, Pages 397–406,

Lassale, C., Batty, G.D., Baghdadli, A. et al. Healthy dietary indices and risk of depressive outcomes: a systematic review and meta-analysis of observational studies. *Molecular Psychiatry* 24, 965–986. 2019

Luders, Eileen et al. "The underlying anatomical correlates of long-term meditation: larger hippocampal and frontal volumes of gray matter." *NeuroImage* vol. 45,3 (2009): 672-8. .2008

Lee, H. et al. "The Efficacy of Hypnotherapy in the Treatment of Irritable Bowel Syndrome: A Systematic Review and Meta-analysis." *Journal of Neurogastroenterology and Motility* vol. 20,2 (2014): 152-62.2014

Leigh, S. "The Rising Popularity of Dance." *SOUK*. 2014. https://www.shoutoutuk.org/2014/09/11/rising-popularity-of-dance-get-involved/

Lemere, C. A., Masliah. E. "Can Alzheimer disease be prevented by amyloid-beta immunotherapy?." *Nature Reviews*. Neurology vol. 6,2. 2010

Leonard, J. "EMDR therapy: Everything you need to know https://www.medicalnewstoday.com/articles/325717 2019

Leslie, M. "The Vexing Legacy of Lewis Terman. The legendary Stanford psychologist helped hundreds of gifted children and showed America that it's okay to be smart. But behind his crusade was a disturbing social vision." *The Stanford Magazine.* 2000

Levine, G., Cohen, B., Commondore-Mensah, Y., et.al. "Scientific Statement From the American Heart Association." On behalf of the American Heart Association Council on Clinical Cardiology; Council on Arteriosclerosis, Thrombosis and Vascular Biology; Council on Cardiovascular and Stroke Nursing; and Council on Lifestyle and Cardiometabolic Healthe, Originally published. 2021

Li, N. et al. "Fecal microbiota transplantation from chronic unpredictable mild stress mice donors affects anxiety-like and depression-like behavior in recipient mice via the gut microbiota-inflammation-brain axis." *Stress* (Amsterdam, Netherlands) vol. 22,5: 592-602. 2019

Limbana, T. et al. "Gut Microbiome and Depression: How Microbes Affect the Way We Think." *Cureus* vol. 12,8 e9966. 23 Aug. 2020

Liu, J., Zhang, Y." Intratumor microbiome in cancer progression: current developments, challenges and future trends." *Biomark Res* 10, 37 2022.

Liu, Hui et al. "Is Sex Good for Your Health? A National Study on Partnered Sexuality and Cardiovascular Risk among Older Men and Women." *Journal of Health and Social Behavior* vol. 57,3: 276-96. 2016

Lopez: Lopez-Garcia, Esther et al. "The relationship of coffee consumption with mortality." *Annals of Internal Medicine* vol. 148,12: 904-14. 2008

MacMahon, B., Yen, S., Trichopoulos, D, et.al. "Coffee and Cancer of the Pancreas. "*N Engl J Med*, 304: 630-633. 1981

Mahmud, N et al. "Increased prevalence of methylenetetrahydrofolate reductase C677T variant in patients with inflammatory bowel disease, and its clinical implications." *Gut* vol. 45,3: 389-94. 1999

Mangeri, Felice et al. "A standard ballroom and Latin dance program to improve fitness and adherence to physical activity in individuals with type 2 diabetes and in obesity." *Diabetology & Metabolic Syndrome* vol. 6 74. 22 Jun. 2014

Marmic, P Mamic, Petra et al. "Gut microbiome - A potential mediator of pathogenesis in heart failure and its comorbidities: State-of-the-art review." Journal of molecular and cellular cardiology vol. 152: 105-117. 2021

Maurier, R. "Music decreases perceived pain for kids in pediatric ER: *U Alberta Medical Research*." University of Alberta. 2013

Mayo Clinic. "Exercise for weight loss: Calories burned in 1 hour." Mayo Clinic. 2020: https://www.mayoclinic.org/healthy-lifestyle/weight-loss/in-depth/exercise/art-20050999

Mayo Clinic. "Exercise for weight loss: Calories burned in 1 hour." Mayo Clinic. 2016

Mayo Clinic. "Insomnia." 2016 https://www.mayoclinic.org/diseases-conditions/insomnia/diagnosis-treatment/drc-20355173

Mayo Clinic. "SAMe" 2020. https://www.mayoclinic.org/drugs-supplements-same/art-20364924

Medicine Mammas. *V Magic*. https://medicinemamasapothecary.com/collections/vmagic 2023

Medline. "Is intelligence determined by genetics?" *Medline Plus*. 2022 https://medlineplus.gov/genetics/understanding/traits/intelligence/

Menon, V. et al. "Vitamin D and Depression: A Critical Appraisal of the Evidence and Future Directions." *Indian Journal of Psychological Medicine* vol. 42,1 11-21. 6 Jan. 2020

Meraii, S., Douglis, S. "Stressed? Instead of distracting yourself, try paying closer attention." *NPR Lifekit*. 2022 https://www.npr.org/2021/12/21/1066585316/mindfulness-meditation-with-john-kabat-zinn

Million Hearts. "Risks for Heart Disease and Stroke." 2019 https://millionhearts.hhs.gov/learn-prevent/risks.html

Mineo, L. "Good genes are nice, but joy is better." *Harvard Gazette.* 2017
https://news.harvard.edu/gazette/story/2017/04/
    over-nearly-80-years-harvard-study-has-been-showing-how-to-
    live-a-healthy-and-happy-life/

Minhas, P.S. Minhas PS, Latif-Hernandez A, et.al. "Restoring metabo-
    lism of myeloid cells reverses cognitive decline in ageing."
    Nature. 2021

Monda, V. et al. "Exercise Modifies the Gut Microbiota with Positive
    Health Effects." *Oxidative Medicine and Cellular Longevity* vol. 2017

Moore, Adam et al. "Regular, brief mindfulness meditation practice
    improves electrophysiological markers of attentional control."
    Frontiers in Human Neuroscience vol. 6 18. 10 Feb. 2012

Morze, J. et al. "An updated systematic review and meta-analysis on
    adherence to Mediterranean diet and risk of cancer." *European
    Journal of Nutrition* vol. 60,3: 1561-1586. 2021

Mozes, A. "Could Good Sex Be Bad for an Older Man's Heart?"
    WebMD. 2016 https://www.webmd.com/healthy-aging/
    news/20160906/could-good-sex-be-bad-for-an-older-mans-heart

Muley A, Muley P, Shah M. "Coffee to reduce risk of type 2 diabetes? :
    a systematic review." *Curr Diabetes Rev.* May;8(3):162-8. 2012

Mursu, J. et al. "Dark chocolate consumption increases HDL choles-
    terol concentration and chocolate fatty acids may inhibit lipid
    peroxidation in healthy humans." *Free Radical Biology &
    Medicine* vol. 37,9: p1351-9. 2004

National Academies Press. "Dietary Reference Intakes for Thiamin,
    Riboflavin, Niacin, Vitamin B6, Folate, Vitamin B12,
    Pantothenic Acid, Biotin, and Choline." 1998 https://www.ncbi.
    nlm.nih.gov/books/NBK114302/.

National Geographic. "Your Amazing Brain." *National Geographic
    Kids.* 2015 https://kids.nationalgeographic.com/science/article/
    your-amazing-brain

NIH: "Major Depression." NIMH. 2022

Nicita-Mauro, V. et al. "Smoking, health and ageing." *Immunity &
    Ageing* : I & A vol. 5 10. 16 Sep. 2008

NIH. "What Are Sleep Deprivation and Deficiency?" *NHLBI* 2022 https://www.nhlbi.nih.gov/health/sleep-deprivation

NIH: "St. John's Wort and Depression: In Depth." *NCCIH*. 2017 https://www.nccih.nih.gov/health/st-johns-wort-and-depression-in-depth https://www.nimh.nih.gov/health/statistics/major-depression#part_2563

NIH. "Parkinson's Disease." NINDS. 2023 www.ninds.nih.gov/health-information/patient-caregiver-education/hope-through-research/parkinsons-disease-hope-through-research

Northwestern Medicine. "11 Fun Facts About Your Brain." *Northwestern Medicine Neurology and Neurosurgery.* 2019 https://www.nm.org/healthbeat/healthy-tips/11-fun-facts-about-your-brain

Northwestern University. "Why Antidepressants Don't Work For So Many." ScienceDaily. ScienceDaily, 27 October 2009.

Novotney, A "Music as Medicine." *Science Watch*. APA. Vol 44(10) p. 46 2013

NSC. "Drivers are Falling Asleep Behind the Wheel." NSC. 2023https://www.nsc.org/road/safety-topics/fatigued-driver?

Nuwar, R. "The World's Happiest Man Is a Tibetan Monk." *The Smithsonian Magazine.* 2012 https://www.smithsonianmag.com/smart-news/the-worlds-happiest-man-is-a-tibetan-monk-105980614/

Pacheko, D. "Deep Sleep: How Much Do You Need?" Sleep Foundation. 2023 https://www.sleepfoundation.org/stages-of-sleep/deep-sleep

Palmer, S. "Fighting Heart Disease, The Dean Ornish Way. *Today's Dietician.* Vol 11 (2) p48. 2009

https://www.todaysdietitian.com/newarchives/td_020909p48.shtml

Panchai: M., Saunders, H,. Rudowitz, R. "The Implications of COVID-19 for Mental Health and Substance Use." *KFF.* 2023 https://www.kff.org/coronavirus-covid-19/issue-brief/the-implications-of-covid-19-for-mental-health-and-substance-use

Parkinson's Foundation. "The Flu Factor: Is There a Link to Parkinson's?" Parkinson's Foundation. 2022 https://www.parkinson.org/blog/science-news/flu

Parkinson's Disease Society. "Drug-induced Parkinsonism." *Information Sheet.* 2008 https://www.parkinsons.org.uk/sites/default/files/2018-09/FS38%20Drug%20induced%20parkinson-ism_0.pdf

Parkinson's Foundation." Deep Brain Stimulation (DBS)." 2023 https://www.parkinson.org/living-with-parkinsons/treatment/surgical-treatment-options/deep-brain-stimulation

Patel AK, Reddy V, Shumway KR, et al. *Physiology, Sleep Stages.* [Updated 2022 Sep 7]. In: StatPearls [Internet]. Treasure Island (FL): StatPearls Publishing; 2022

Peirce, D. "Music is Physical – The Importance of Exercise for Musicians." *Physiotec.* 2021

Penckofer, S. et al. "Vitamin D Supplementation Improves Mood in Women with Type 2 Diabetes." *Journal of Diabetes Research* vol. 2017

Penetar, D., McCann, U., Thorne, D., et. al. "Effects of Caffeine on Cognitive Performance, Mood, and Alertness in Sleep-Deprived Humans." *NIH.* 1994 https://www.ncbi.nlm.nih.gov/books/NBK209050/

Perez, A. "9 Health Benefits of Lion's Mane Mushroom (Plus Side Effects)." *Healthline,* 2023 https://www.healthline.com/nutrition/lions-mane-mushroom

Pileggi, C., Blondin, D., Hooks, B., "Exercise training enhances muscle mitochondrial metabolism in diet-resistant obesity." *Lancet.* Vol 83 (104192) 2022

Pinniger, Rosa et al. "Argentine tango dance compared to mindfulness meditation and a waiting-list control: a randomised trial for treating depression." *Complementary Therapies in Medicine* vol. 20,6: 377-84 2012

Powers, R. "Use It or Lose It: Dancing Makes You Smarter, longer." *Stanford Dance.*2010

Prabhakaran,D .,Anard, S., Gaziano, TA. et. al. *Cardiovascular, Respiratory, and Related Disorders*. 3rd edition. Washington (DC): The International Bank for Reconstruction and Development / The World Bank; 2017 Nov 17.

PTSD. "Eye Movement Desensitization and Reprocessing (EMDR) Therapy." *APA*. 2023 https://www.apa.org/ptsd-guideline/ treatments/eye-movement-reprocessing

Quinlan, C. "The Importance of Learning Something New As You Age." Metro Health. 2016 https://metrohealthinc.com/2016/08/31/ the-importance-of-learning-something-new-as-you-age/

Raghaven, S., Vassy, J.,Ho, Y., et. al. "Diabetes Mellitus-Related All-Cause and Cardiovascular Mortality in a National Cohort of Adults." *JAHA* Vol 8. 2019 https://www.ahajournals.org/ doi/10.1161/JAHA.118.011295

Ray, F. "Dancing the Tango May Reduce Fall Risk, Help With Balance." *Parkinson's News Today*. 2021

Reza, J., Van Heel, D. 46-A Magical Number. *Health and Genes.* 2023 https://www.genesandhealth.org/ genes-your-health/46-%E2%80%93-magical-number

Richards, T. *Overcoming Social Anxiety: Step by Step*. Create Space Independent Publishing Platform. 306 pages. 2014 https://www. amazon.com/Overcoming-Social-Anxiety-Step/dp/1497584566

Rose, C. *Neurology of Music*. World Scientific Publishing Co. 2010 https://books.google.com/books?id=xDnICgAAQBAJ&pg=PA21 &lpg=PA21&dq=%E2%80%

Ruhl, T. " Napoleon Dynamite: A conversation with Jon Heder." Victory Theatre 2022 https://usishield.com/37495/features/ napoleon-dynamite-a-conversation-with-jon-heder-efren- ramirez-jon-gries-was-surprisingly-inspirational-and-irresist- ibly-fun/

Rutkowski K, Sowa P, Rutkowska-Talipska J, Kuryliszyn-Moskal A, Rutkowski R. Dehydroepiandrosterone (DHEA): hypes and hopes. *Drugs*. 2014 Jul;74(11):1195-207. doi: 10.1007/s40265-014- 0259-8. PMID: 25022952.

Salas, J., Bullo, M, Babio, N., et. al. "Reduction in the Incidence of Type 2 Diabetes With the Mediterranean Diet." *Diabetes Care.* 34:14-19, 2011 https://www.ncbi.nlm.nih.gov/pmc/articles/PMC3005482/pdf/zdc14.pdf

Sarris, J et al. "Omega-3 for bipolar disorder: meta-analyses of use in mania and bipolar depression." *The Journal of Clinical Psychiatry* vol. 73,1. 2012

Schmit, S. L., et al. "Coffee Consumption and the Risk of Colorectal Cancer." *Cancer Epidemiology, Biomarkers & Prevention:* a publication of the American Association for Cancer Research, cosponsored by the American Society of Preventive Oncology vol. 25,4: 634-9. 2016

Schnitzler, P et al. "Melissa officinalis oil affects infectivity of enveloped herpesviruses." *Phytomedicine : International Journal of Phytotherapy and Phytopharmacology* vol. 15,9 (2008): 734-40.2008

Schönenberger, K. A., et al. "Effect of Anti-Inflammatory Diets on Pain in Rheumatoid Arthritis: A Systematic Review and Meta-Analysis." *Nutrients* vol. 13,12 4221. 24 Nov. 2021

Schwarcz, J. "What are Endorphins?" *McGill.* 2017 https://www.mcgill.ca/oss/article/you-asked/what-are-endorphins

Science Learning. Mitochondria-Cell Powerhouses. *Science Learning Hub.* 2023 https://www.sciencelearn.org.nz/resources/1839-mitochondria-cell-powerhouses

Seidler, R. D et al. "Motor control and aging: links to age-related brain structural, functional, and biochemical effects." *Neuroscience and Biobehavioral Reviews* vol. 34,5: 721-33. 2010

Seppälä, J. et al. "Association between vitamin b12 levels and melancholic depressive symptoms: a Finnish population-based study." *BMC Psychiatry* vol. 13 145. 24 May. 2013, doi:10.1186/1471-244X-13-145

Shaw, G. "Aphasia Won't Stop Gabby Giffords from Speaking Out. Gabby Giffords doesn't let aphasia stop her from speaking out on behalf of others with the condition." *Brain & Life.* 2022 https://www.brainandlife.org/articles/gabby-giffords-doesnt-let-aphasia-stop-her

Shelton, R. C., et al. "Assessing Effects of l-Methylfolate in Depression Management: Results of a Real-World Patient Experience Trial." *The Primary Care Companion for CNS Disorders* vol. 15,4. 2013

Shoichet, C. "Tony Bennett, 95, leaves his heart on stage in a moving final concert with Lady Gaga. *CNN Entertainment.* 2021. https://www.cnn.com/2021/11/28/entertainment/tony-bennett-lady-gaga-concert/index.html

Siddiqui, M., and Cresci, G. "The Immunomodulatory Functions of Butyrate." *Journal of Inflammation Research* vol. 14 6025-6041. 18 Nov. 2021

Siebern, A. T., et al. "Non-pharmacological treatment of insomnia." *Neurotherapeutics : the journal of the American Society for Experimental NeuroTherapeutics* vol. 9,4: 717-27. 2012

Smith, B. "8 Health Benefits of Having an Orgasm." M&F. 2023 https://www.muscleandfitness.com/women/sex-tips/8-health-benefits-having-orgasm/

Smithers, L., Golley, R., Mittinty, M., et. al. "Dietary Patterns at 6,15, and 24 months of age are associated with IQ at 8 years of age. *European Journal of Epidemiology.* 27, 525-535. 2012

Snowdon DA; Nun Study. Healthy aging and dementia: findings from the Nun Study. *Ann Intern Med.* Sep 2;139(5 Pt 2):450-4. 2003

Stamatakis E, Ekelund U, Ding D, Hamer M, Bauman AE, Lee IM. "Is the time right for quantitative public health guidelines on sitting? A narrative review of sedentary behavior research paradigms and findings". *Br J Sports Med.* 2019 Mar;53(6):377-382. 2019

Stanford. The New Map of Life. *Stanford Medicine.* 2023. https://longevity.stanford.edu/the-new-map-of-life-report/

Statista: "Share of adults who watch more online exercise videos due to social distancing during the coronavirus pandemic in the United States as of March 26, 2020." 2022. https://www.statista.com/statistics/1108538online-fitness-video-usage-during-coronavirus-usa/

Stewart, A.H., Wallentin, L., Benatar, J., et.al. "Dietary patterns and the risk of major adverse cardiovascular events in a global study of high-risk patients with stable coronary heart disease." *European Heart Journal*, Volume 37, Issue 25, Pages 1993-2001. 2016

Stulberg D, Ewigman B. Antidepressants causing sexual problems? Give her Viagra. *J Fam Pract.* 57(12):793-6. 2008

Sweet, L. 365 *Sex Positions: A New Way Every Day for a Steamy, Erotic Year*, July 7, 2020 Amorata Press. 376 pages

Tankslamen, A., Hibbein, J., Tuomilehto, J. et.al. "Fish Consumption and Depressive Symptoms in the General Population in Finland." *APA*. Apri,2001 https://doi.org/10.1176/appi. ps.52.4.529

Teixeira, Diogo S et al. "Enjoyment as a Predictor of Exercise Habit, Intention to Continue Exercising, and Exercise Frequency: The Intensity Traits Discrepancy Moderation Role." *Frontiers in Psychology* vol. 13 780059. 18 Feb. 2022

Thimbleby, Harold. "Technology and the future of healthcare." Journal of Public Health Research vol. 2,3 e28. 1 Dec. 2013

Thomson, Blake et al. "Association Between Smoking, Smoking Cessation, and Mortality by Race, Ethnicity, and Sex Among US Adults." *JAMA* network open vol. 5,10 e2231480. 3 Oct. 2022

Tinsley, G. "6 Benefits of Reishi Mushroom (Plus Side Effects and Dosage)." *Healthline*, 2023 https://www.healthline.com/ nutrition/reishi-mushroom-benefits

Toledo E, Salas-Salvadó J, Donat-Vargas C, et al. Mediterranean Diet and Invasive Breast Cancer Risk Among Women at High Cardiovascular Risk in the PREDIMED Trial: A Randomized Clinical Trial. *JAMA Intern Med.*:175(11) 2015

Torres, L. "'Napoleon Dynamite' star Jon Heder reveals his iconic dance scene was almost set to a Michael Jackson song and other behind-the-scenes secrets." *Insider.* 2021 https://www.insider. com/napoleon-dynamite-dance-scene-jon-heder-jamiro- quai-2021-6

Trafton, A. "Unique visual stimulation may be new treatment for Alzheimer's. Noninvasive technique reduces beta amyloid plaques in mouse models of Alzheimer's disease." *MIT News.* 2016. https://news.mit.edu/2016/visual-stimulation-treatment-alzheimer-1207

Trimble, M. "U.S. Kids More Likely to Die Than Kids in 19 Other Nations The U.S. could have spared 600,000 lives if it kept pace with other wealthy nations, a study finds." *US News.* 2018 https://www.usnews.com/news/best-countries/articles/2018-01- 11/us-has-highest-child-mortality-rate-of-20-rich-countries.

University of Alabama. "Gut Microbiome at the Center of Parkinson's Disease Pathogenesis." *Neuroscience News.* 2022 https://neurosciencenews.com/gut-microbiome-parkinsons-21981/

UC Davis. "Paleo diet: What it is and why it's not for everyone." *UC Davis News.* 2022 https://health.ucdavis.edu/blog/good-food/paleo-diet-what-it-is-and-why-its-not-for-everyone/2022/04

Ursell, Luke K et al. "Defining the human microbiome." *Nutrition Reviews* vol. 70 Suppl 1,Suppl 1: S38-44. 2012. Vallance, J., et al. "Evaluating the Evidence on Sitting, Smoking, and Health: Is Sitting Really the New Smoking?" *American Journal of Public Health* vol. 108,11: 1478-1482. 2018

Van Dyck, C., Swanson, C., Aisen, P., et. al. "Lecanemab in Early Alzheimer's Disease." *N Engl J Med* 388:9-21. 2023 https://www.nejm.org/doi/full/10.1056/NEJMoa2212948

Vargas-Soria, M., Carranza-Naval, M., Marco, A., et. al. "Role of liraglutide in Alzheimer's disease pathology." *Alzheimer's Research and Therapy.* 2021 https://alzres.biomedcentral.com/articles/10.1186/s13195-021-00853-0

Verghese, J., Lipton, R, Katz, M., et. al. "Leisure Activities and the Risk of Dementia in the Elderly." *N Engl J Med*;348:2508-2516. 2003

Vielle, R. "Neurofeedback Can Raise Your IQ Scores? Really?" *Monterey Bay Neurofeedback.* 2019 https://www.montereybayneurofeedback.com/post/question-you-can-use-neurofeedback-training-to-raise-iq-scores-really

Wan, L., Li, Y., Zhang, Z. et al. Methylenetetrahydrofolate reductase and psychiatric diseases. *Transl Psychiatry* 8, 242. 2018

Wan, Minjie et al. "Serotonin: A Potent Immune Cell Modulator in Autoimmune Diseases." *Frontiers in Immunology* vol. 11 186. 11 Feb. 2020

Wani, Ab Latif et al. "Omega-3 fatty acids and the treatment of depression: a review of scientific evidence." *Integrative Medicine Research* vol. 4,3: 132-141.2015

Warren, T., et al. "Sedentary behaviors increase risk of cardiovascular disease mortality in men." *Medicine and Science in Sports and Exercise* vol. 42,5): 879-85.

W, K. "45 Orgasm Statistics Are Better When They're About Orgasms" *Pleasure Better.* 2022. https://pleasurebetter.com/orgasm-statistics/#References

Weeks, John. "Integrative MEND Protocol for Reversing Alzheimer's Picked Up in Aging and by George Washington University … plus more." *Integrative Medicine* (Encinitas, Calif.) vol. 15,4: 24-6. 2016

Weiler, Marina et al. "Transcranial Magnetic Stimulation in Alzheimer's Disease: Are We Ready?" *eNeuro* vol. 7,1 ENEURO.0235-19.2019. 7 Jan. 2020, doi:10.1523 / ENEURO.0235-19.2019

Wenger: Buijsse, Brian et al. "Cocoa intake, blood pressure, and cardiovascular mortality: the Zutphen Elderly Study." Archives of internal medicine vol. 166,4: 411-7. 2006

Whelton P, Carey R, Aronow W, et al. 2017 ACC/AHA/AAPA/ABC/ACPM/AGS/APhA/ASH/ASPC/NMA/PCNA Guideline for the Prevention, Detection, Evaluation, and Management of High Blood Pressure in Adults. J Am Coll Cardiol. May, 71 (19) e127–e248. 2018

Whiteman, W. "Coffee consumption linked with reduced melanoma risk." Medical News Today. 2015https://www.medicalnewstoday.com/articles/288316

Williams, B. "What Percentage of Gym Memberships Go Unused?" Exercise.Com. 2021. https://www.exercise.com/learn/unused-gym-memberships-percentage

Williams, Stefanie et al. "Eating chocolate can significantly protect the skin from UV light." *Journal of Cosmetic Dermatology* vol. 8,3: 169-73. 2009

Wilson, D. "Everything You Should Know About Maitake Mushroom." *Healthline.* 2017 https://www.healthline.com/health/food-nutrition/maitake-mushroom

Woei Hwang PW, Braun KL. The Effectiveness of Dance Interventions to Improve Older Adults' Health: A Systematic Literature Review. *Altern Ther Health Med.* 2015 Sep-Oct;21(5):64-70. 2015

Wong, Kah-Hui et al. "Peripheral Nerve Regeneration Following Crush Injury to Rat Peroneal Nerve by Aqueous Extract of Medicinal Mushroom Hericium erinaceus (Bull.: Fr) Pers. (Aphyllophoromycetideae)." Evidence-based complementary and alternative medicine: eCAM vol. 2011. 2011

World Dance Sport Federation. "Fit Through Dance." 2023. https://www.worlddancesport.org/About/All/Fit_Through_Dance

Wu, R., Strickland, C. "Think You're Too Old to Learn New Tricks?" *Scientific American.* 2019. https://blogs.scientificamerican.com/observations/think-youre-too-old-to-learn-new-tricks/

Wu, S.i et al. "Nonexercise physical activity and inflammatory and oxidative stress markers in women." Journal of women's health. vol. 23,2: 159-67. 2002

Xue, L., Yang, X., Tong, Q., et.al. "Fecal microbiota transplantation therapy for Parkinson's disease." *Medicine* (99)35. 2020 https://journals.lww.com/md-journal/fulltext/2020/08280/fecal_microbiota_transplantation_therapy_for.103.aspx

Yang, B. et al. "Effects of regulating intestinal microbiota on anxiety symptoms: A systematic review." *General Psychiatry* vol. 32,2 e100056. 17 May. 2019

Yarnall, C., Qian, X. "Older Adult Playfulness." AJP. 2011: https://files.eric.ed.gov/fulltext/EJ985548.pdf

YouTube. https://www.youtube.com/watch?v=yRnb7vor-oQ. Rafi Eldor *Dance Through Life* video. 2016

Yuan S, Li X, Jin Y, Lu J. "Chocolate Consumption and Risk of Coronary Heart Disease, Stroke, and Diabetes: A Meta-Analysis of Prospective Studies." *Nutrients*. 2;9(7):688. 2017

Zagursky, E. "It's not all in your head — it's in your gut, too." William and Mary News. 2015, https://www.wm.edu/news/stories/2015/fermented-food-social-anxiety-study123.php

Zhang, Q. et al. "Metformin therapy and cognitive dysfunction in patients with type 2 diabetes: A meta-analysis and systematic review." *Medicine* vol. 99,10. 2020

Zhang, Y. et al. "Consumption of coffee and tea and risk of developing stroke, dementia, and poststroke dementia: A cohort study in the UK Biobank." *PLoS Medicine* vol. 18,11 e1003830. 16 Nov. 2021,

Zieglestein, C. "How Depression and Heart Disease Relate to Each Other." *Johns Hopkins Medicine*. 2023 https://www.hopkinsmedicine.org/health/conditions-and-diseases/depression-and-heart-disease

Zullo J., Drake, D., Aron, L., et. al. "Regulation of lifespan by neural excitation and REST." 2019. https://www.nature.com/articles/s41586-019-1647-8